Comparing and Contrasting the Impact of the COVID-19 Pandemic in the European Union

```
T0384401
```

Comparing and Contrasting the Impact of the COVID-19 Pandemic in the European Union challenges the use of uncontextualised comparisons of COVID-19 cases and deaths in member states during the period when Europe was the epicentre of the pandemic. This timely study looks behind the headlines and the statistics to demonstrate the value for knowledge exchange and policy learning of comparisons that are founded on an in-depth understanding of key socio-demographic and public health indicators within their policy settings. The book adopts innovative, integrated, multi-disciplinary international perspectives to track and assess a fast-moving topical subject in an accessible format. It offers a template for analysing policy responses to the COVID-19 pandemic and for using evidence-based comparisons to inform and support policy development.

Linda Hantrais FAcSS is Emeritus Professor of European Social Policy at Loughborough University, UK, and a Visiting Professor at the London School of Economics and Political Science. Her research interests span international comparative research theory, methods, management and practice, with particular reference to public policy and institutional structures in the European Union, and the relationship between socio-demographic trends and social policy.

Marie-Thérèse Letablier is Senior Research Fellow at the Centre National de la Recherche Scientifique (CNRS), and Emeritus Senior Research Fellow at the Centre d'Economie de la Sorbonne-UMR 8174, Université Paris 1 Panthéon-Sorbonne. Her research focusses on family policy, intergenerational relations and the work–family relationship in France, from an international comparative perspective.

Routledge Studies in Political Sociology

For a full list of titles in this series, please visit: https://www.routledge.com/
sociology/series/RSPS

Comparing and Contrasting the Impact of the COVID-19 Pandemic in the European Union

Linda Hantrais and
Marie-Thérèse Letablier

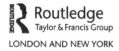

Routledge
Taylor & Francis Group

LONDON AND NEW YORK

First published 2021
by Routledge
2 Park Square, Milton Park, Abingdon, Oxon OX14 4RN

and by Routledge
605 Third Avenue, New York, NY 10017

First issued in paperback 2022

Routledge is an imprint of the Taylor & Francis Group, an informa business

Publisher's Note
The publisher has gone to great lengths to ensure the quality of this
reprint but points out that some imperfections in the original copies
may be apparent.

British Library Cataloguing-in-Publication Data
A catalogue record for this book is available from the British Library

Library of Congress Cataloging-in-Publication Data
A catalog record has been requested for this book

ISBN: 978-0-367-69175-2 (pbk)
ISBN: 978-0-367-69172-1 (hbk)
ISBN: 978-1-003-14071-9 (ebk)

DOI: 10.4324/9781003140719

Typeset in Times New Roman
by codeMantra

Contents

Figures

Tables

Boxes

Notes on the authors

Linda Hantrais is a Fellow of the UK Academy of Social Sciences, Emeritus Professor of European Social Policy at Loughborough University, UK, and a Visiting Professor at the London School of Economics and Political Science. Her research interests span international comparative research theory, methods, management and practice, with particular reference to public policy and institutional structures in the European Union, and the relationship between socio-demographic trends and social policy. She has coordinated several European research projects on these topics. Her publications include *Social Policy in the European Union* (2007), *International Comparative Research: Theory, Methods and Practice* (2009) and *What Brexit Means for EU and UK Social Policy* (2019).

Marie-Thérèse Letablier is Senior Research Fellow, Centre National de la Recherche Scientifique (CNRS), and Emeritus Senior Research Fellow, Centre d'Economie de la Sorbonne-UMR 8174, Université Paris 1 Panthéon-Sorbonne. She was formerly a research associate at the Institut national d'études démographiques (Ined), Paris, and is currently a member of the Haut Conseil de la Famille, de l'Enfance et de l'Age. She has participated in several European research projects and networks, and she has acted as a policy adviser for research programmes in Japan and South Korea. Her research interests encompass intergenerational relations, family, childcare, family–work reconciliation and gender equality policies. She has published widely on these topics with a particular focus on family solidarities in France and Europe.

Preface

On 13 March 2020, the World Health Organisation (WHO, 2020d) officially recognised Europe as the epicentre of the COVID-19 pandemic. The media and politicians used information about absolute numbers of cases and deaths from the virus in European Union (EU) member states to construct league tables and to identify best policy practice for curbing the spread and severity of the pandemic. In combination, under-reporting, under-diagnosis and missing cases were known to create serious limitations for statisticians and data users, thereby undermining the value of comparisons made without reference to their sources or to the diverse socio-demographic, economic and political contexts within Europe (Hantrais, 2020b).

The starting point for this book was the decision to challenge the inappropriate and misleading use of comparisons of the impact of the pandemic in EU member states. The chapters look behind the headlines and statistics to demonstrate the value for knowledge exchange and policy learning of comparisons of COVID-19 cases and deaths founded on an in-depth understanding of key socio-demographic and public health indicators within their policy settings. Using evidence-based comparisons, the authors adopt multi-disciplinary international perspectives to track the progress of the pandemic across the EU and to assess the strengths and weaknesses of the policymaking process.

Finding the right distance for comparisons

According to the principle of 'variable distance' (*verschiedene Distanz*), developed by Georg Simmel (1917) over a century ago, the distance of the analyst from the object under observation affects the way it is observed and conceptualised. The long-distance perspective can be exemplified in the European context by the innumerable reports published by the EU, based on data collated by the Commission's statistical agency (Eurostat), and on published statistics collated and analysed by the many international organisations and research institutes cited in this book. Of necessity, these reports are mainly confined to description, since their primary purpose is to provide snapshots of situations based on aggregated statistics in a large number of countries for a limited number of variables at a given point in time.

By contrast, a close-up or granular comparison of a social phenomenon, such as the COVID-19 pandemic, within a country or region, can reveal differences that may not be apparent when aggregated national-level data are being compared from a distance. The close-up view allows identification, as exemplified in this book, of variations in key socio-demographic and health indicators, and policy environments. These factors may result in greater disparities within societies or cultures than between them. A combination of the long and close perspectives is of greatest value when studying the impact of COVID-19 in the EU, since most public health policy is framed at national or supranational levels, while responsibility for implementation is delegated to subnational authorities, resulting in regional and local disparities.

The implications of any changes in the mix or number of countries and the level of analysis may be the addition of less similar units of observation. Any shift in focus affects both the findings and their interpretation. Within the EU, the six waves of enlargement altered the European 'mean'. They changed territorial boundaries and the cultural and linguistic mix, giving the lie to much received wisdom (Hantrais, 2007).

If the focus of the book were to be enlarged to encompass more nation states and continents – China, India, the Americas, South Korea or Japan, for example – what emerge as significant differences within and between EU member states would pale into insignificance. A different set of contextual factors would need to be incorporated to achieve meaningful comparisons. The framework adopted in this book could serve as a template for such studies.

The European Union as a framing device

All member states are subject to the same supranational legislative framework as a condition of membership of the Union. Public health is an area of policy where national governments have retained responsibility for making and implementing decisions. But heads of state and government are also involved in determining EU-level policy. Since the 1992 Maastricht Treaty (Article 129), the EU has had a public health mandate. EU institutions are charged with ensuring a high level of human health protection, with coordinating action between member states and cooperation with them to prevent diseases and combat cross-border threats to health. Maastricht made explicit the EU's remit to promote research into the causes and transmission of 'major health scourges'. The 2007 Lisbon Treaty (Article 168) conceded that 'Union action shall respect the responsibilities of the Member States for the definition of their health policy and for the organisation and delivery of health services and medical care'.

The fact that nation states retain responsibility for formulating, organising and delivering their own public health policy means that EU-wide comparisons are rarely comparing like with like. The varied reactions of societies to the global pandemic highlight the complexities of the task assigned to EU institutions in coordinating national policy responses and formulating policy recommendations that would be acceptable to all governments and to their electorates.

The aim of the study was to investigate the impacts of the pandemic across EU member states prior to and during the months – February to July 2020 – when Europe was the epicentre of the crisis and in the immediate aftermath. This approach made an already complex task even more complicated because the pandemic raised issues about the capacity and willingness of EU member states to cooperate with EU institutions. The temptation was compelling for heads of state and governments to self-isolate and to give priority, amid conflicting pressures, to protecting what they considered to be the national interest. The same argument applied within countries: local and regional administrations took the initiative in applying restrictive measures to suppress local outbreaks of the disease. The European Commission struggled to carry out its treaty commitments in the public health area, while respecting the competence of EU member states to decide and deliver public health policies. Nor did it want to lose sight of its global positioning and the role it intended to play in driving climate change policy.

A further complication was the lack of complete, reliable and comparable datasets about the spread of the virus during the period under study. Although member states receive instructions for compiling information according to common definitions and standards, national statistical offices and other administrative bodies are not always willing or able to observe these requirements. Consequently, data sources and methods of collection, case definitions, recording and reporting practices vary both within and between countries. Data collected before the onset of the pandemic provided some indication of public healthcare capacity, but they were of limited value in measuring the readiness of individual countries to deal with a major health scourge. The analysis had to rely on a combination of data harvested from a variety of sources to build a picture of the impact of COVID-19 across the EU and of national policy responses.

During the pandemic, experts were called upon to advise governments. Scientists from all disciplines were rarely in agreement, but data journalists and politicians at EU and national levels constantly referred to what was described as the 'best scientific evidence available' to compare the speed and extent of the introduction of protective measures across and within countries. Drawing on examples of 'best practice' from elsewhere, the media and opposition politicians used international comparisons, often between neighbouring EU member states, to highlight the shortcomings and bottlenecks of policies introduced by their own governments.

The EU has made many attempts over the years to achieve closer social union, but major differences persist both in the organisation and financing of national public health systems, and in methods of delivery and performance. The distribution and partial sharing of competences in the public health area, therefore, proved to be problematic in managing the COVID-19 pandemic. National governments did not wait for directions from Europe before assuming responsibility for introducing their own restrictive measures to contain the spread of the disease. They consistently flouted EU rules on state aid, free movement of goods and people across borders, public procurement and debt limits. Progressively, the European Commission was galvanised into easing restrictive legislation. It deployed its public health remit to monitor and coordinate the actions taken by individual member states and to encourage cooperation in easing lockdown and planning economic recovery. Whether, in the longer term, the pandemic will have exacerbated divisions or brought nations closer together in a struggle against a common (invisible) enemy remains to be seen.

Linda Hantrais and Marie-Thérèse Letablier
London and Paris
September 2020

1 European national public healthcare systems compared

This chapter presents the socio-economic and public health settings within which coronavirus was to reach pandemic proportions. It begins with a review of public health data sources and their limitations before examining the reliability and comparability of the data collected in different socio-demographic, economic and political contexts. The chapter demonstrates the importance of situating comparisons in relation not only to key demographic indicators (population size, density and age distribution, and household composition), but also to the socio-economic environments in which national health systems are embedded. Both healthcare status and the capacity to prevent and react to health emergencies are examined. The review covers funding arrangements, levels of expenditure, provision of hospital and institutional care beds, various aspects of medical capacity, interventions to prevent diseases and preparedness to deal with public health emergencies. The conclusion considers how, in combination, socio-demographic characteristics and public health indicators can contribute to the comparative analysis of the impacts of COVID-19 in different policy settings.

Public health data sources and their limitations

Despite attempts throughout the EU's history to harmonise social provisions, major differences have persisted not only in the overall level of state spending per capita on social protection and the structure of contributions, but also in methods of delivery and performance of national systems (Hantrais, 2007, 2019, 2020a). Problems of comparability and reliability associated with public health data both over time and across countries often seem intractable. Media coverage of the pandemic is prone to look for the best or worst performing countries on selected indicators. The inference is that practices adopted in other countries could serve as models. However, the league tables compiled by data journalists rarely comment on the reasons why policy responses might be effective in a specific societal context, and why they may, or may not, be transferable to different socio-economic and political settings.

A plethora of data are available to track and monitor the social situation across the EU in the early 21st century. Eurostat, the EU's statistical office, regularly collects and collates national data based, as far as possible, on the same definitions and standards, and covering the same time periods. In the healthcare area, the EU has established a set of 88 European Core Health Indicators (ECHI) providing a comprehensive knowledge system of allegedly comparable health data for use in monitoring health and informing policymaking at EU level (European Commission, n.d.a, n.d.b). These indicators map demographic characteristics and socio-economic situations in EU member states. They cover health status, including causes of death, the incidence of selected communicable diseases and healthy life expectancy; determinants of health; and health interventions, extending across service provision, expenditures on health and health promotion policies. Since 1990, the EU's Mutual Information System on Social Protection (MISSOC, 2020) collates annually updated, detailed information supplied by government departments in member states about national legislation, benefits and conditions. MISSOC provides separate tables for healthcare and sickness cash benefits.

In recognition of national diversity in social rights, in 2016 the European Commission (n.d.c) established a Social Scoreboard designed to track the comparative performance of member states. The Commission uses the Scoreboard as a 'screening device' and monitoring tool to enable wider assessment of the social situation in individual member states. The Scoreboard focusses on comparative data in three areas: equal opportunities and access to the labour market; dynamic labour markets and fair working conditions; and public support/social protection and inclusion. This last category includes a section on healthcare, presenting indicators for self-reported unmet need for medical care; healthy life years at the age of 65; and out-of-pocket expenditure on healthcare.

Together these sources provide comprehensive, though not always complete or very recent, datasets on public healthcare that can be used to situate and contextualise the responses of national governments to COVID-19. When used for comparative purposes, contextual data about health systems come with many of the same caveats as indicators of the spread of the pandemic and the policy measures introduced to deal with it (Chapters 2 and 3). Although countries are instructed to compile ECHI information using common definitions and criteria, national statistical offices are not always able or willing to observe these instructions due to the non-availability of certain data and variations in sources and methods of collection.

Obstacles such as these result in under-reporting, under-diagnosis and missing data. In a report on the state of health in the EU, OECD/European Union (2018, pp. 100, 102, 114, 126, 170) refer to numerous data limitations. Under-reporting is, for example, estimated to be as high as 40% in the case of HIV and tuberculosis. Caution is advised in presenting and interpreting cases of vaccine-preventable diseases due to diversity in surveillance systems, case definitions and reporting practices. In recording the prevalence of diseases, some countries collect data on acute but not chronic cases. Furthermore, variations between countries may reflect differences in testing, immunisation and screening programmes, as well as sample size and data collection methods. Where self-reporting is used in surveys, for instance to measure healthy life expectancy or unmet medical need, extra caution is required since subjective assessments may be influenced by socio-cultural factors. Reported causes of death vary considerably both between and within countries, as was starkly revealed during the pandemic (Chapter 2). Variations may be explained by the capacity to test for the virus, differences in medical protocols, coding practices and death certification processes, as well as the presence of underlying life-threatening conditions, and the account taken of the setting in which deaths occur. The failure to situate the number of deaths in relation to socio-demographic factors (population size, density and age distribution, gender, ethnicity, living and working conditions) further distorts the picture provided by daily trend figures.

An additional problem in contextualising daily information about cases and deaths across the EU during the pandemic is that full datasets, such as those prepared by ECHI, take time to complete and to check and are often published after several years' delay. For example, the most recent European-wide data on public health laboratory capacity available when the crisis began dated from 2016; indicators for the number of curative hospital care beds or unmet need in relation to population size referred to 2017; complete datasets were not available at EU level with information about residential care homes. Data that can be accessed provide an indication of potential preparedness, but they do not record the actual capacity to deal with a major health crisis when it strikes. More useful comparative data must be sought by tracking the capacity of health services to scale up provision in the weeks following the outbreak of the disease. The numbers of excess deaths directly and indirectly attributable to the pandemic provide a better indication of the pandemic's impact, but they may only be known sometime after the event when governments are being held to account for their actions, or they may never be known.

Public health in socio-demographic contexts

In selecting contextual indicators that might be helpful in situating and interpreting information about COVID-19 cases and deaths as well as policy measures to control and treat the disease, this section focusses on socio-demographic and public health data based on internationally agreed definitions and collection methods. Due reference is made to the caution that must be exercised if these data are to have any explanatory value.

Demographic statistics

Comparisons of the number of COVID-2019 cases and deaths reported on a given date, or during a specified period, are often made without reference

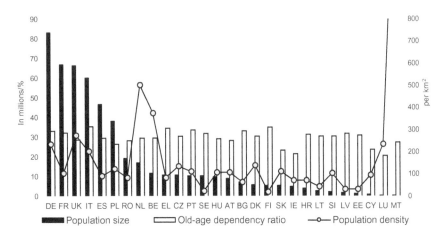

Figure 1.1 Demographic statistics.
Sources: Eurostat (n.d.e): old-age-dependency ratio (% of total population aged over 65), 2019; Eurostat (n.d.g): population density (km²), 2018; Eurostat (n.d.h): population size (millions), 2019.

to the corresponding population size, density or age distribution. These fundamental demographic data might be expected to influence observations, as can be illustrated using Eurostat demographic statistics for the 28 EU member states in pre-pandemic years (Figure 1.1).

Six countries comprise between 38 (Poland) and 83 (Germany) million inhabitants (left axis), and 15 between 0.5 (Malta) and 9.8 (Hungary) million. Population density (right axis) ranges from 18 (Finland) to 1,548 (Malta) inhabitants per square kilometre. Old-age-dependency ratios (% of total population aged over 65, left axis) range between 20.7 (Luxembourg) and 35.7 (Italy).

All things being equal, large countries (Germany, France, the UK, Italy and Spain) would be expected to report many more cases of infections and deaths in absolute numbers than small countries (Slovenia, Lithuania, Latvia, Estonia, Cyprus, Luxembourg and Malta). Alternatively, population density might be a more influential factor, in which case the Netherlands, Belgium and the two small island states, Malta and Cyprus, would be expected to record relatively high rates of infection and COVID-19 deaths. Large urban agglomerations (London, Paris, the Ruhr, Madrid) might also be expected to register large numbers of cases and deaths as they become hotspots due to both their size and population density. Infections are known to be more likely to result in death among older people, who are, in turn, more likely to have underlying health conditions. The implication is that countries with high old-age-dependency ratios (Italy, Finland, Greece and Portugal) would be expected to record relatively high rates. In Chapter 2, these predictions are tested with reference to absolute and relative figures for COVID-19 cases and deaths.

Public health expenditure

The extent to which demographic factors may be mitigated by public health policy can be assessed by comparing selected healthcare indicators. An important difference between member states concerns the ways in which public health systems are funded and structured (Figure 1.2).

Eurostat data for the years prior to the outbreak of the pandemic show that expenditure on health as a proportion of GDP fell in most EU28 member states. Between 2010 and 2018, the decline was most marked in Ireland, Greece and Lithuania, whereas the increase was greatest in Croatia. All member states spent more on health than on education, where expenditure also fell over the same period. The Irish case may be explained by the significant increase in GDP in 2015 when some big economic operators relocated to Ireland, resulting in a substantial reduction in the proportion of GDP spent on social protection (OECD/European Union, 2018, p. 134). Despite these changing patterns, the same countries remained at each end of the scale: Denmark, Austria and France spent the largest proportion of their GDP on health in 2018, and Romania, Latvia and Cyprus the smallest proportion.

When adjusted to take account of differences in price levels between EU member states, per capita spending on health in purchasing power standards (PPS) was highest in Germany, Luxembourg, Sweden and the Netherlands in 2017; it was lowest in Romania, Latvia, Bulgaria and Croatia.

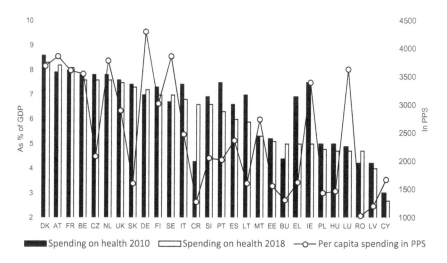

Figure 1.2 Public health expenditure.

Sources: Eurostat (n.d.c): expenditure on health (% GDP), 2010/2018; Eurostat (2020b, table 1): per capita spending (in PPS), 2017.

The relatively high figure for Luxembourg is explained by the fact that a large proportion of workers contributing to GDP are non-residents and are, therefore, excluded from the per capita figures. The level of spending on health per capita is relevant in the context of the pandemic in that higher spending might be expected to be associated with higher recovery rates from diseases and lower case fatality rates (the total number of deaths as a proportion of reported cases).

Information about the ways in which healthcare is funded and the proportion of GDP devoted to healthcare are indicative of both the level of support provided by the state and the way in which resources are managed (Figure 1.3, left axis). Government schemes contributed over 70% of funding for healthcare in Denmark, Sweden, the UK, Italy and Ireland in 2017. In Luxembourg, Germany, France, Slovakia, Croatia and the Netherlands, 75% or more of funding depended on compulsory contributory insurance schemes. In Cyprus, Bulgaria and Latvia, over 40% of funding was raised from other sources.

MISSOC tables for Health Care in 2020 show that government schemes are usually funded from general taxation and are conditional on legal/permanent residence. Insurance schemes involve varying levels of contributions from employers, employees and the self-employed as well as government subsidies. In addition, countries with decentralised or devolved healthcare systems (Germany, Italy, Spain and the UK) display regional differentiation in healthcare decision-making and delivery, which may hamper comparisons of data at national level, but which may help to explain how some national governments delegated responsibility for implementing COVID-19 measures adapted to meet local needs.

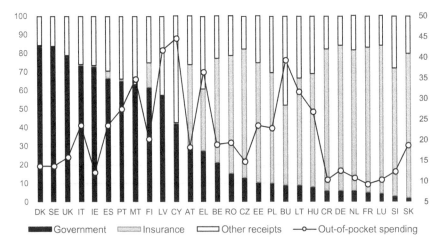

Figure 1.3 Healthcare funding sources and out-of-pocket spending.
Sources: Eurostat (n.d.f): out-of-pocket spending (as % of total health expenditure), 2019; Eurostat (2020b, p. 9): healthcare funding by source (in %).

Out-of-pocket payments are expenditures (as a % of all current health expenditure) borne directly by patients from primary income or savings, where payment is made by the user when the goods or services are purchased (Figure 1.3, right axis). A much larger proportion of the cost is borne out of people's own pockets in Bulgaria, Cyprus and Latvia, the countries showing the largest proportions of funding from other sources. By contrast, out-of-pocket expenditure is relatively low in France, Luxembourg, Croatia and the Netherlands, where funding depends primarily on compulsory insurance systems; often provision is made for supplementary cover in return for contributions to optional schemes. In addition, most EU member states provide basic treatment free of charge to categories of resident citizens living below subsistence level (MISSOC, 2020).

Healthcare resources and capacity

Several of the ECHI indicators provide information about health status, determinants and interventions, from which a picture can be built of everyday healthcare needs and the capacity of health systems to deal with emergencies. The Social Scoreboard indicator for healthy life years at age 65 combines information on mortality and morbidity to measure the number of years that a person at age 65 is expected to live in a healthy condition, defined as the absence of disability (OECD/European Union, 2018, p. 86). The rates displayed in the graph (Figure 1.4) suggest that the Central and Eastern European member states might be expected to record relatively high death rates in their older population during the pandemic due to their lower healthy life expectancies. Although the differences between men and

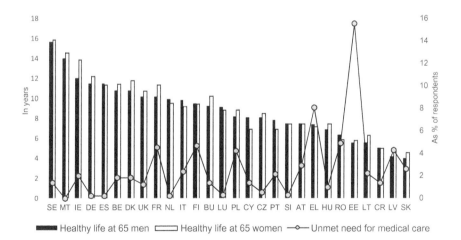

Figure 1.4 Health status.
Sources: Eurostat (n.d.d): healthy life years at age 65 by sex, 2018/2019; Eurostat (n.d.i): self-reported unmet need for medical care (% of respondents), 2018/2019.

women were small in most countries, in 16 cases, women were found to enjoy more healthy life years at age 65. The largest differences in favour of men were observed in Romania, Italy, Portugal and Luxembourg. Where women outlived men, they usually did so by a larger number of years.

The ECHI indicators for self-reported unmet need for medical care rely on information from the European Statistics on Income and Living Conditions (EU-SILC) survey and refer to unmet needs during the previous 12 months (Figure 1.4). This indicator is subject to the usual caveats about the limited comparability of survey questions, sampling issues and self-reporting. Data are expressed as percentages within the population aged 16 and over living in private households. Respondents were asked whether they thought they needed examination or treatment by a specific type of healthcare service (excluding dental treatment), but did not seek it or did not receive it for 'financial reasons', 'waiting list' or 'too far to travel'. In seven countries, unmet need was reported by less than 1% of respondents. Estonia and Greece reported the highest levels. Provided that data collection issues are accounted for, the unmet need indicator could be of interest in assessing the collateral effect of rationing medical treatment for patients suffering from other life-threatening chronic and acute diseases during the pandemic.

Public healthcare systems are known to vary in their capacity to meet medical needs and in the uptake of provisions (Figure 1.5). Preventable mortality is defined as causes of death that can be avoided through effective public health and primary prevention interventions before the onset of diseases/injuries to reduce their incidence. Data available for 2017 (left axis) suggest that France, the Netherlands, Italy and Sweden were, at that time,

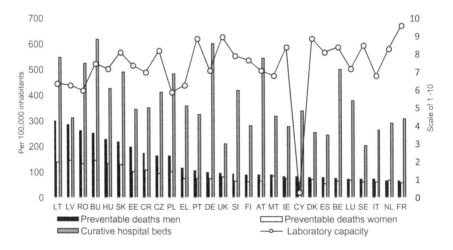

Figure 1.5 Public healthcare protective capacity.

Sources: Eurostat (n.d.b): curative care beds in hospitals (per 100,000 inhabitants), 2018; Eurostat (n.d.j): treatable and preventable mortality (men and women per 100,000 inhabitants), 2017; OECD/European Union (2018, p. 197): public health laboratory capacities (scores 1–10), 2016.

most successful in preventing premature deaths, whereas Lithuania, Latvia, Romania, Bulgaria and Hungary were least successful in doing so. Avoidable deaths were due mainly to heart disease and alcohol-related illnesses and were most prevalent among men, suggesting why men might be more likely than women to die if they contract the virus.

Since hospital care accounts for more than half of expenditure on health, the number of curative care beds in relation to population size provides an indication of the resources available for delivering services to inpatients. The data are, however, not directly comparable because some countries exclude psychiatric and private sector beds (OECD, 2019a, p. 194). Since 2000, the number of beds per capita has been decreasing in most EU member states. By 2016, the largest reduction occurred in Finland, where the fall was over 50%, mainly affecting long-term care beds and psychiatric care beds. Part of the decrease can be attributed to advances in medical technology, allowing more surgery to be performed on a same-day basis, or as part of a broader policy strategy to reduce the number of hospital admissions.

Data for 2017 (Figure 1.5) indicate that Germany, Bulgaria, Austria and Hungary possessed the largest number of curative care beds in hospitals per 100,000 inhabitants, whereas Italy, Spain, Denmark, Ireland, the UK and Sweden – countries with national health services – had gone furthest in reducing the number of beds. They also tended to be the countries aiming at relatively high occupancy rates (Eurostat, n.d.a, 2020e). Low availability of curative (acute) care beds was to become a major source of concern during the pandemic.

Another indicator of the preparedness of countries to deal with pandemics is their laboratory capacity (Figure 1.5). Data for this indicator are derived from EULabCap monitoring surveys carried out annually in EU member states. The surveys are conducted to assess the resilience of health systems and their ability to detect emerging diseases accurately in time to stop outbreaks. The EULabCap's composite index comprises 60 technical indicators of laboratory structure with 10 as the maximum score (right axis). The data are subject to several limitations: some indicators vary due to differences in national systems, self-reporting of data and technological innovations (OECD/European Union, 2018, p. 196). Data for 2016 suggest that France, the UK, Portugal, Denmark and Sweden were best prepared at that time, whereas Italy, Greece and Poland were among the laggards.

Information about other healthcare resources in earlier years shows that medical goods constituted the second largest function in 2017 after curative care (Eurostat, 2020b, p. 7). Member states varied substantially in the proportion of expenditure devoted to this budget head. The lowest shares (below 15%) were recorded for Finland, Ireland, Luxembourg, Sweden, the Netherlands and Denmark. By contrast, the highest shares, where medical goods accounted for between 30% and 35% of current healthcare expenditure, were recorded for Hungary, Greece, Latvia and Slovakia, with a peak at 43% in Bulgaria.

In addition to the capacity to provide intensive care hospital beds, medical equipment, testing facilities and personal protective equipment (PPE), an important factor in ensuring the preparedness of health services to respond to a public health crisis is the availability of appropriately trained medical and nursing personnel support staff (Figure 1.6). Information about practising physicians and nurses is included in the ECHI indicators for healthcare resources. OECD/European Union (2018, p. 178) define practising physicians as doctors who are providing care for patients. Some countries include doctors working in administration, management, academic and research positions, as well as interns and doctors in training, described as 'professionally active' physicians (another 5–10% of doctors). Greece and Portugal report all physicians entitled to practise, resulting in an over-estimation. In Belgium, a minimum threshold of activities (500 consultations per year) is set for general practitioners to be considered as practising, resulting in an under-estimation compared with countries that do not set a minimum threshold.

The number of medical doctors per 100,000 population is relatively stable across member states: highest in Greece and Austria and lowest in Poland, the UK and Luxembourg. Traditionally, in most EU member states, the medical profession, particularly in the higher ranks, has been male dominated. A Eurostat (2020d, figure 4) analysis for 2017 showed that the proportion of female physicians had generally increased between 2007 and 2017: 15 member states reported that women were in the majority. In Estonia and Latvia, more than 80% of physicians were women. Men continued to account for over 60% of physicians in Luxembourg and Cyprus.

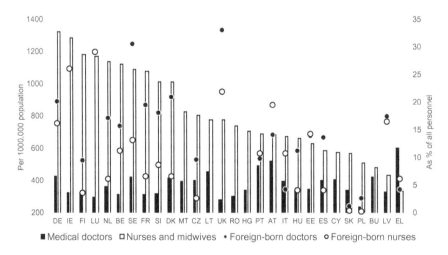

Figure 1.6 Healthcare personnel.
Sources: Eurostat (n.d.i, 2020c): medical doctors, nurses and midwives (per 100,000 inhabitants), 2018; OECD (2019b, p. 17): foreign-born doctors, nurses (as % of all doctors, nurses), 2015/16.

OECD/European Union (2018, p. 180) define practising nurses as those providing services for patients in public and private settings, but they point out that some countries include managers, educators or researchers. The data may distinguish between different levels of nursing: 'professional' nurses (general and specialist nurses) and 'associate professional' nurses who have a lower level of qualifications. In addition, Austria and Greece are found to report only nurses working in hospitals resulting in an under-estimation. Germany and Ireland record the highest figures for nurses, while the positions for Greece and Luxembourg are the reverse. Although the gender of nurses is not reported in the Eurostat statistics, women are believed to account for more than 80%.

As the pandemic spread, the impact of the virus on different population groups of frontline workers became an issue of concern. OECD (2019b, figures 1.3 and 1.4) provide information about foreign-born doctors and nurses. Their data covered 22 EU member states and referred to 2015/2016. At that time, Ireland and the UK displayed the largest proportions of foreign-born doctors and nurses, and Poland and Slovakia the smallest proportions. The OECD report does not specify the countries from where foreign-born medical personnel come, although they note that the largest proportion of foreign-trained doctors in Ireland were found to have trained in Pakistan. In the UK, nearly a third of all foreign-trained doctors in 2017 came from India, followed by 11% from Pakistan (OECD, 2019b, p. 33). Data for the UK indicate that, in 2020, the most common nationalities in the Nation Health Service, other than British, were Indian, Filipino, and Irish, and that the numbers from EU member states had fallen since the 2016 referendum, whereas the number of non-EU nationals had increased (House of Commons Library, 2020).

Long-term institutional and informal care provision

The very high death rates of older people in residential care homes drew attention to the poor provision of long-term care. The European Pillar of Social Rights (European Commission, 2017) had identified access to affordable and good quality long-term care services as one of its core principles. A European Social Policy Network's (ESPN) study found that the EU's rapidly ageing societies were facing similar challenges in long-term care (European Commission, 2018). The emphasis in the ESPN study was on community-based care: nursing and residential provision in specially designed facilities or hospital-like settings was recognised as a necessary complement for people with moderate to severe functional restrictions.

ESPN showed that provision in Europe was characterised by significant differences in organisation, delivery and financing of residential care, both between and within countries, resulting in fragmentation of responsibilities and the lack of integration between health and social aspects (European Commission, 2018, pp. 6–9). The authors found that, in many countries

(Denmark, Finland, the Netherlands and Sweden), the supply of residential care facilities for older people had been reduced in line with policies aimed at deinstitutionalisation, whereas elsewhere the trend was in the opposite direction due to the decline in the availability of informal carers (Italy, Spain and Portugal). The situation was more mixed in the Central and Eastern European member states, with declining institutional care in some countries (Latvia), and an increase in the number of residential homes in others (Bulgaria, Estonia, Lithuania and Romania). A private commercial sector had developed to cater for the demand among those who could afford to pay for it (Cyprus, Greece, Hungary, Malta, Portugal, Romania and the UK). The financial crisis resulted in cuts in public funds and the tightening of eligibility criteria for state provision in some countries (Croatia, Denmark, Greece, Spain, Ireland and the UK).

Only long-term care that relates to the management of the deterioration in a person's health is usually reported as health expenditure, although it is difficult, in certain countries, to separate out the health and social aspects of long-term care (OECD/European Union, 2018, p. 136). The most recent available data for expenditure on long-term healthcare (as distinct from social care), both as a percentage of all spending on health and as a percentage of GDP, suggest that, in 2017, Sweden, the Netherlands, Denmark and Belgium were spending more on long-term care than Bulgaria, Romania and Greece (Figure 1.7). The number of long-term care beds are also difficult to compare. Several countries only include beds in publicly funded facilities, while others also include private facilities (both for-profit and not-for-profit).

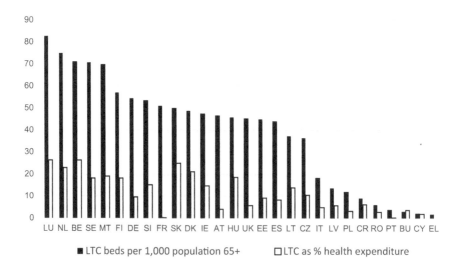

■ LTC beds per 1,000 population 65+   ☐ LTC as % health expenditure

Figure 1.7 Long-term care provision.

Sources: Eurostat (2020b, table 6): long-term care (as % of expenditure on health), 2017; OECD (2019a, figure 11.26): long-term care beds in institutions per 1,000 population aged 65 and over, 2017.

Some countries count beds in treatment centres for addicted people, psychiatric units of general or specialised hospitals, and rehabilitation centres.

Cross-country comparisons of care-home provision are highly unreliable, as demonstrated by attempts to record and compare deaths from COVID-19 other than in hospital settings (Chapter 3). More reliable data are needed to distinguish between: deaths of older people who are transferred to hospital after having contracted COVID-19 in a residential care home and subsequently die in hospital; deaths that occur within the care home without transfer to a hospital; and deaths in care homes for patients with other conditions requiring hospital care, who have been discharged from hospitals to care homes to free up beds. In all cases, higher proportions of COVID-19-related death might be expected among care-home residents than in the wider population of the same age, since frail elderly people are most likely to be in care homes, and care-home residents are most likely to display underlying conditions and to be most vulnerable to infection in the care setting.

Data for the amount of informal care provided by family members are, by definition, difficult to access. In Hungary, Latvia and Lithuania, family responsibilities of children for their parents are enshrined in law, including the obligation to contribute to the cost of care for elderly parents in residential care homes. Various benefits in cash and kind are available to support carers (European Commission, 2018, pp. 7, 17–18).

Eurostat data for family composition indicate that growing proportions of the population are living alone, particularly in Denmark, Finland and Sweden, Germany and Estonia (Figure 1.8). The share of older people living

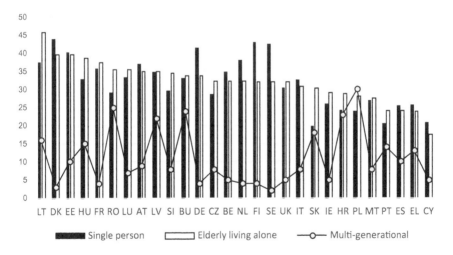

Figure 1.8 Household composition.
Sources: Eurostat (2017): share of the elderly living alone, 2017; Eurostat (n.d.b): single-person households (as % of households), 2018; Verbist et al. (2020, figure 1): multi-generational households (as % of households), 2013.

alone is high in Denmark and Estonia, as well as in Latvia, Hungary and France. Recent data for all EU member states are not available for the number of multi-generational households. Earlier data show that coresidence of generations was more common in most Central and Eastern European than in the Nordic countries (Figure 1.8). A study of 11 EU member states suggests that the higher prevalence of intergenerational coresidence in southern European countries associated with later transition to adulthood increases the likelihood of COVID-19 transmissions from younger to older generations (Ehl et al., 2020).

The combined impact of demographic characteristics and public health policy settings

The analyses in this chapter suggest that political decision-takers could usefully consider the possible impact of various combinations of socio-demographic and public health indicators on the numbers of cases and deaths during the COVID-19 epidemic. Figure 1.9 combines cumulative data for selected demographic indicators (population size, density and age

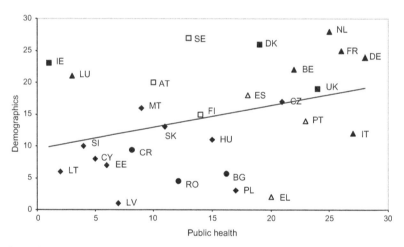

Legend :

▲ Wave 1 Belgium, France, Germany, Italy, Luxembourg, Netherlands

■ Wave 2 Denmark, Ireland, UK

△ Wave 3 Greece, Portugal, Spain

□ Wave 4 Austria, Finland, Sweden

◆ Wave 5 Czechia, Cyprus, Estonia, Hungary, Latvia, Lithuania, Malta, Poland, Slovakia, Slovenia

● Wave 6 Bulgaria, Croatia, Romania

Figure 1.9 Risk factors in public health policy settings.
Source: Authors' compilation from data in Figures 1.1–1.8.

distribution), and associated potential 'risk' factors, with information about national public health policy settings (per capita spending on health and long-term care, unmet need, laboratory, personnel, hospital and residential care bed capacity) as potential factors contributing to and mitigating risks. Chapters 2–5 build on the multiplicity of factors reviewed in this chapter to gain a better understanding of the comparative value of this patterning for the analysis of COVID-19 infection and death rates.

2 Comparing the impacts of COVID-19 across EU member states

This chapter scrutinises the data available about the spread of COVID-19 across EU member states during the period when Europe was at the epicentre of the pandemic. The chapter begins by examining the different definitions and methodologies used to collect and collate data on the numbers of COVID-19 cases and deaths. It identifies issues of data reliability and comparability. Analysis of compilations of full datasets for EU member states illustrates how the positioning of different countries in league tables varies as a result of differences in recording and reporting practices. An assessment based on the limited data available about excess deaths by age illustrates the impact of COVID-19 on mortality rates over time. Reference is made to the debate in the scientific community about the value of the R (reproduction) number and K (dispersion) factor in estimating the rate of transmission of the disease when used to assist policymakers in deciding whether to strengthen or ease lockdown. The conclusion considers to what extent expectations about the spread of COVID-19, based on socio-demographic indicators and information about the capacity of national public health systems, match the outcomes observed.

Issues of COVID-19 data reliability and comparability

After a delay of several weeks, the World Health Organisation (WHO, 2020d) announced that Europe had become the epicentre of the pandemic. The misuse of comparisons between EU member states of absolute numbers of COVID-19-related deaths became widespread in the media, to the extent that scientists and statisticians warned against making cross-country comparisons (Donnelly, 2020; Spiegelhalter, 2020). Data gathered at international level by Eurostat or one of the institutions tracking and reporting worldwide trends can only be as good as the information supplied at national and local levels. When member states join the EU, their statisticians receive training from Eurostat in data collection and analysis to ensure that their returns meet EU requirements. In early 2020, Eurostat (2020a) issued practical guidance for national statistical offices on the methodological issues triggered by COVID-19 regarding the collection of standard socio-demographic and economic data during the pandemic. Their guidelines included advice on how to conduct routine surveys – Labour Force Surveys, EU-Statistics on Income and Living Conditions (EU-SILC), national accounts data and metadata – using alternatives to face-to-face interviews.

COVID-19 data sources

Eurostat did not gather and process their own data on COVID-19 infections and deaths in EU member states. In this chapter, alternative widely cited online data sources are used extensively to track and report different dimensions of COVID-19 cases and deaths (Box 2.1).

Box 2.1 International COVID-19 data sources

Worldometer (n.d.a), an international team of developers, researchers and volunteers, based in the US, aim to make world statistics available 'in a thought-provoking and time relevant format'. They offer a valuable live source of information about the daily situation worldwide, which can be sorted by region. Their category for 'Europe' includes EU member states, except Cyprus, and they specify that they 'work to ensure ... data is protected in accordance with applicable EU laws'. Their daily updates are recognised as being relatively reliable and unbiased and are used by the John Hopkins University Center for Systems Science and Engineering (Donovan, 2020), and extensively by data journalists at Politico EU and other national and international news agencies, including the BBC, Deutsche Welle, *Financial Times*, *Economist* and *Le Monde*.

   Our World in Data (n.d.), based at the Oxford Martin Programme on Global Development, is a scientific online web tool, founded in 2011 by Max Roser, a social historian and development economist. His team focusses on large global problems. They make available daily updated research and data about the pandemic. They also publish articles that use multifactorial methods to look behind the statistics.

   Politico EU (n.d.a, n.d.b) is a global nonpartisan politics and policy news organisation with offices in Brussels, London, Berlin, Paris, Rome and Warsaw, through which it 'connects the dots between global power centers'. Since 1 March 2020, Politico EU has provided a live coronavirus data tracker specifically for EU member states and the UK.

   Since 2008, the European Commission's European Mortality Monitoring collaborative network (EuroMOMO, 2020a, 2020b), located in Denmark, has been tasked with undertaking a European mortality monitoring activity, supported by the European Centre for Disease

Prevention and Control (ECDC) and WHO. In 2016, the network began using a European statistical model based on pooled data from 24 European countries or regions to produce graphs and maps showing the weekly total number of excess deaths for all ages and for different age groups. The network covers 16 EU member states, Norway and Switzerland. Only Berlin is included for Germany, and data are recorded separately for England, Northern Ireland, Scotland and Wales. EuroMOMO's aim is to calculate the causes of mortality and excess morbidity related to seasonal influenza, pandemics and other public health threats. They use Z-scores to measure the standard deviation of deaths enabling comparisons to be made between different populations and time periods (EuroMOMO, 2020c). In their data, excess mortality rates above 15 are considered to be extremely high.

The network advises that, in its graphs for COVID-19 excess deaths,

> the number of deaths shown for the three most recent weeks should be interpreted with caution, as adjustments for delayed registrations may be imprecise. Furthermore, results of pooled analyses may vary depending on countries included in the weekly analyses. Pooled analyses are adjusted for variation between the included countries and for differences in the local delay in reporting.
>
> (EuroMOMO, 2020a)

It further cautions that 'the network hub is not mandated by the participating countries to release any national data', thereby limiting the value of the tool for comparative analyses.

Aron & Muellbauer (2020), both researchers at the Institute for New Economic Thinking, Oxford University, argue that interpreting large differences in excess mortality between countries requires consideration of three main factors, and the within-nation deviations in these factors: the average infection rates in preceding weeks, average mortality risk from COVID-19 and constraints on COVID-19-specific health capacity. They recommend using P-scores to aid comparability: P-scores define excess deaths as deviations from 'normal' deaths plus a margin adjusting for the uncertainty of excess mortality statistics within countries by age groups, city size and occupational, social and ethnic groups.

The Care Policy and Evaluation Centre (CPEC) at the London School of Economics conducted a regularly updated study focussing specifically on mortality associated with COVID-19 outbreaks among residents in care homes (Comas-Herrera et al., 2020). The CPEC team collated and analysed data on mortality in 14 EU member states and in the regions of the UK, supplied by 'trusted' national informants.

Defining COVID-19 cases and deaths

Chapter 1 reviewed many of the reasons why countries do not always follow closely instructions issued by international agencies when compiling national statistics. These problems were exacerbated in the case of the pandemic by the demand from governments for the most-up-to-date daily figures with which to track the number of infections and deaths and inform policy. Decision-takers need to ensure an adequate supply of tests, personal protective equipment, ventilators, hospital beds and trained staff. Published information about the number of COVID-19 deaths occurring daily in EU member states are, however, of limited value for international comparisons due in large part to discrepancies in the clinical and biological criteria used to identify the cause of death, the place where it occurred and the time period covered.

Worldometer are careful to define deaths and to alert users to issues of reliability and comparability in the statistics they produce. When they refer to total cases, they mean the reported

> total cumulative count of detected and laboratory (and sometimes, depending on the country reporting them and the criteria adopted at the time, also clinically) confirmed positive and sometimes − depending on the country reporting standards − also presumptive, suspect, or probable cases of detected infection. Because it represents a cumulative count (rather than a snapshot of the number of current cases at any given time), this number can't decrease. The size of the gap between detected (whether confirmed, suspect or probable) and reported cases versus actual cases will depend on the number of tests performed and on the country's transparency in reporting. Most estimates have put the number of undetected cases at several multiples of detected cases.
>
> (Worldometer, n.d.c)

They list the number of 'Active Cases' as total cases minus total deaths and recoveries. This statistic represents 'the current number of people detected and confirmed to be infected with the virus' and serves as 'an important metric for Public Health and Emergency response authorities when assessing hospitalization needs versus capacity'. They acknowledge that the statistic for recoveries is

> highly imperfect, because reporting can be missing, incomplete, incorrect, based on different definitions, or dated (or a combination of all of these) for many governments, both at the local and national level, sometimes with differences between states within the same country or counties within the same state.
>
> In some countries, when a patient is discharged from the hospital it [sic] is counted as 'recovered' even if no test is performed. Some health

officials now consider anyone who was diagnosed with COVID-19 three or more weeks ago and has not died to be recovered from the disease. In view of this, 'Active Cases' and 'Closed Cases Outcome' which both depend on the number of recoveries (in addition to an accurate death count and a satisfactory rate of case detection, both of which are lacking in the vast majority of countries) can be affected by this inherent flaw for many countries and for the total worldwide count.

(Worldometer, n.d.c)

The descriptor 'Serious and Critical' in the tables is also deemed to be 'imperfect' for many of the same reasons. According to Worldometer, 'it represents for the most part the number of patients currently being treated in [an] Intensive Care Unit (ICU), if and when this figure is reported'.

These definitional issues are compounded, as noted by Worldometer, when the number of deaths is being recorded on specific days due to 'official governmental channels changing or retracting figures or publishing contradictory data on different official outlets'. Worldometer keep 'a log with a partial list of errors, retractions, or major discrepancies (and their explanation) between our numbers and what users could see on other outlets'. In May 2020, for example, when a spike had been passed in most EU member states, they found discrepancies in data reported for France, Ireland, Italy and Spain.

Recording and reporting COVID-19 tests, infections and deaths

Scrutiny of information about data collection and reporting practices in individual member states reveals many more examples that help to explain why international comparisons of daily figures are of limited value. Statistics for tests, cases and deaths vary markedly depending on the data source (registry of deaths, national statistical office, research institute) and the frequency of recording and reporting (daily or weekly) (Box 2.2).

Box 2.2 National statistical sources and data collection methodologies

A common feature in EU member states is their use of a combination of national statistical offices, government departments, agencies and research institutes to track and analyse the characteristics of cases in their populations. National statistical offices generally collect and process mortality figures, based on deaths registered at local level. In principle, these data provide full, weekly counts of all deaths associated with COVID-19. Methods of collection and reporting vary both within and between countries. They take time to compile and are normally published between a week and a fortnight after the end of the week in which the deaths occurred.

Government departments for health and other agencies are tasked with collecting real-time data on COVID-19 infections and deaths to provide a snapshot of what is happening day-by-day in their health and care systems. They record the numbers of deaths occurring daily in hospitals, though not necessarily on the same day. For example, deaths during the weekend may not be reported until the following week. Nor do the daily counts always report deaths that occur in residential care homes or in the community, since these data are collected at local level from a variety of uncoordinated sources.

During the pandemic, the French Institut national d'études démographiques (Ined, 2020) carried out a regularly updated, fully documented analysis of COVID-19 deaths in seven EU member states: Denmark, France, Germany, Italy, the Netherlands, Portugal, Spain, and England and Wales. Their documentation illustrated the methodological issues and the resulting discrepancies in daily cumulative death counts arising from different testing regimes and the place where deaths were recorded. In most of the countries studied, initially in March 2020, they found that COVID-19 tested deaths in hospitals were the primary, and most reliable, source of daily counts.

In addition to the numbers of cases and deaths, Worldometer and Our World in Data provide statistics for the number of COVID-19 tests performed in each country to detect the presence of the virus. The European Commission (2020, 18 March) issued recommendations to EU member states for testing strategies, including prioritising tests for patients in hospitals and care homes with underlying respiratory infections and other chronic medical conditions. They advised on the different means that could be used to conserve resources but did not refer to the link that might be made between testing and the numbers of COVID-19-related deaths.

Doubts have been cast on the accuracy and reliability of virus testing, particularly as used in the early phases of the pandemic. Tests were, for example, found to produce both false negatives and false positives. The lack of reliable tests, and the limited number of authorised testing centres and laboratories affected the number of tests that could be carried out and the population groups able to access them. Testing strategies varied from one country to another owing mainly to the limited availability of test kits and laboratory capacity, as well as the time taken by laboratories to analyse tests. Some governments chose to test their entire populations; others focussed on suspect cases with few symptoms; others only tested their health professionals and individuals with severe symptoms. As a result, many of the COVID-19 deaths reported may not have been accurately attributed to the disease. Cases may also have been missed in the cumulative counts since the statistics could not be corrected at a later date. Countries gradually built up capacity, enabling them to extend eligibility for testing to different categories of the population, from hospital staff and patients to those in residential homes, and from symptomatic to asymptomatic cases.

The Ined (2020) study showed that, from the outset, Germany's Robert Koch-Institut, as the sole data collection source in Germany, was recording all tested COVID-19 deaths wherever they occurred, albeit with a few days delay. Denmark also reported all tested deaths wherever they occurred. The Netherlands were reporting tested deaths in hospitals and elsewhere, but in the knowledge that not all patients were being tested.

A second COVID-19 test was not widely available during the first wave of the pandemic to detect antibodies built up as part of the immune response to disease due to past infection. Whereas virus testing could be used for diagnosis of COVID-19, an antibody test was sought for information about the spread of the virus within the population (UK Research and Innovation, UKRI, 2020), and the extent of its containment when governments were planning their lockdown exit strategies (Chapter 3).

Establishing the cause of death is problematic. It may be certified by biological tests, clinical diagnosis and by mentioning the disease on the death certificate. In many countries, the first results based on daily figures concerned only hospital deaths. Patients who died in hospital were generally tested before death, but deaths in institutions or in the patient's home could be suspected, but not proven, to be associated with COVID-19. In both cases, the virus may have been the major cause, a contributory factor or simply present when a person was dying of something else (Oke & Henegan, 2020). Both frequency of testing and the place where deaths are recorded (hospital, care home, community) are, therefore, important factors contributing to variations in daily counts between countries and over time, making it difficult, if not impossible, to compile consistent datasets at a specific point in time within or across countries.

Measuring the spread and impact of the pandemic

Scientists monitoring the progression of the pandemic have adopted what is commonly known as the 'reproduction number' (R) to track the transmission of the disease and, thereby, to assist policymakers in monitoring its spread (Box 2.3).

Box 2.3 The reproduction number (R) and dispersion factor (K)

Scientists at Imperial College London (ICL) and the London School of Hygiene and Tropical Medicine (LSHTM) in the UK, at the Institut national d'études démographiques (Ined) and Institut national de la santé et de la recherche médicale (Inserm) in France, and the Robert Koch-Institute (RKI) in Germany have developed models for measuring the spread of the virus. When R is higher than 1, the number of cumulative cases is increasing exponentially. At 3 the spread of the disease is deemed to be out of control, which was the situation in many EU member states reporting large numbers of cases and deaths during March and April 2020.

Why some COVID-19 patients infect many others, whereas most patients do not spread the virus at all, has puzzled scientists. The dispersion factor (K) has been suggested as an alternative to R to describe how much a disease 'clusters', to identify super-spreaders and to assess how COVID-19 is transmitted. The lower the K, the more transmission comes from a small number of people or an event (super-spreaders), enabling targeted efforts to be made to control an outbreak. Scientists have estimated that only 10–20% of COVID-19 infected people are responsible for 80% of transmissions, whereas 70% of those infected may not transmit the virus at all (Aget, 2020; Kupferschmidt, 2020).

The reproduction number, and modelling more generally, has been criticised for using inappropriate paradigms and assumptions, such as the 1918 influenza pandemic or, more recently, the SARS epidemic in 2002–03, and the 2009 influenza virus, to determine rates of transmissibility, clinical severity and community spread, as well as the age groups most affected (Adam, 2020).

The intractable issues involved in accurately monitoring the number of COVID-19 infections and deaths on a daily basis, or even ten or more days later, complicate attempts to compare national data. Many experts therefore counsel adopting a different approach enabling the calculation of excess deaths directly or indirectly attributable to the virus (Robine, 2020). Analysts may then be in a better position to gauge whether the virus is bringing forward deaths by a few months for people who are known to be nearing the end of their life (Triggle, 2020).

WHO define 'excess mortality' as:

Mortality above what would be expected based on the non-crisis mortality rate in the population of interest. Excess mortality is thus mortality that is attributable to the crisis conditions. It can be expressed as a rate (the difference between observed and non-crisis mortality rates), or as a total number of excess deaths.

(WHO, n.d.b)

Excess mortality for a given period is calculated from the number of people who died during the period compared to the number who would have been expected to die from all causes based on the same period in previous years (Ritchie et al., 2020). Excess mortality data include 'collateral damage' from other health conditions if the health system is overwhelmed by COVID-19 cases. Scientists have suggested that additional deaths could be related to people being deterred from seeking treatment for medical emergencies such as strokes or heart attacks, and from delaying routine operations and cancer screening. Conditions such as mental health problems and suicides linked to self-isolation, heart problems from lack of activity, the impact on health from increased unemployment and reduced living standards are likely to contribute to excess mortality in the aftermath of the pandemic.

Excess mortality data overcome two problems in reporting COVID-19-related deaths: miscounting attributable to misdiagnosis and under-reporting (EuroMOMO, 2020b; Krelle et al., 2020). However, few countries have statistical agencies with the capacity and infrastructure to report the number of people who died day-to-day, in a given week or even month, over a period of several years. For those that do, excess death rates can offer a valuable tool for making meaningful cross-country comparisons of COVID-19's direct and indirect impact without having to rely on accurate statistics for the number of proven COVID-19-related deaths.

Tracking COVID-19 infections and deaths

By 13 March 2020, more cases and deaths were being reported in Europe than in the rest of the world combined, except for China (Worldometer, n.d.b). This section draws on data from a combination of sources to track the spread of the virus across and within EU member states, with a focus on deaths in care homes and excess mortality.

Timing of cases and death

The first confirmed COVID-19 cases in the EU were recorded in France on 24 January 2020, although a suspect pneumonia case was reported there on 27 December 2019. All EU member states reported their first cases between 24 January and 9 March. By mid-March rates were soaring in Italy, Spain and France, but not all EU member states had reported their third confirmed COVID-19 death. By late April, daily numbers of cases and deaths had peaked, and the pandemic was moving on to other parts of the world.

After France, the first EU member states to report cases were Germany, Finland, Italy, Spain, Sweden and the UK (Table 2.1). Third deaths were first reported in Italy, France, Spain, the Netherlands, the UK, Germany and Belgium. Among these countries, the Netherlands displayed the shortest time lag between the two dates, joined by Ireland, whereas Finland and Sweden recorded the longest interval. In addition, Finland was late in reporting its third death.

When information about the relationship between the dates of the first cases and third deaths is set within the context of statistics showing the absolute number of cases and deaths recorded on 1 April 2020, Spain, Italy, France, the UK and Belgium were the countries recording the largest

Table 2.1 First cases, third deaths and days between cases and deaths

Country	1st case	3rd death	Days cases–deaths	1 April 2020 Confirmed cases	Confirmed deaths
Austria	25 February	17 March	21	10182	128
Belgium	4 February	12 March	37	16982	1305
Bulgaria	8 March	19 March	11	399	8
Croatia	25 February	26 March	30	867	6
Cyprus	9 March	25 March	16	262	8
Czechia	1 March	25 March	24	3308	31
Denmark	27 February	16 March	18	2860	90
Estonia	27 February	30 March	32	745	4
Finland	28 January	28 March	60	1384	17
France	24 January	3 March	39	52128	3523
Germany	27 January	12 March	45	67366	732
Greece	26 February	15 March	18	1314	49
Hungary	4 March	21 March	17	525	20
Ireland	29 February	15 March	15	3235	71
Italy	31 January	25 February	25	105792	12430
Latvia	2 March	11 April	40	398	0
Lithuania	28 February	25 March	26	533	7
Luxembourg	29 February	19 March	19	2178	23
Malta	7 March	11 April	35	184	0
Netherlands	27 February	9 March	11	12595	1039
Poland	4 March	15 March	11	2311	33
Portugal	2 March	20 March	18	7443	160
Romania	26 February	22 March	25	2245	69
Slovakia	6 March	15 April	40	363	0
Slovenia	4 March	23 April	50	814	13
Spain	31 January	6 March	35	111680	8189
Sweden	31 January	16 March	45	4435	180
UK	31 January	9 March	38	33954	2426

Sources: Our World in Data (2020b, 2020c): cases and deaths at 1 April 2020; Politico EU (n.d.b): third deaths; Wikipedia (n.d.b): first cases.

number of deaths on that date (primarily in hospitals), signalling their position at the core of the epicentre. They had all been among the first countries to register first cases and third deaths but with different time lags. At the other end of the scale, almost all the countries recording low numbers of cases and deaths on 1 April also reported later onsets of the disease and some of the largest gaps between the dates of first cases and third deaths.

The positions of countries at the two ends of the scale were confirmed as the pandemic progressed. This patterning might be explained, at least in part, by discrepancies in testing and recording practices, as well as delays between symptom onset and deaths. Almost all the countries reporting the highest/lowest numbers of cases and deaths were characterised in Chapter 1 as member states with the largest/smallest population sizes and/or highest densities.

Comparing daily and cumulative cases, deaths and tests

As countries reached and passed the peaks in the numbers of deaths and began preparing to exit lockdown in mid-May (Chapter 3), governments monitored closely daily updates of the cumulative statistics for infections, deaths and tests in their own and other countries (Table 2.2). Only absolute numbers of cases and deaths at 1 April are presented in Table 2.1. Table 2.2 displays absolute and relative numbers (per million inhabitants) of cases, deaths and tests at 17 May to illustrate the importance of situating statistics in relation to population size if comparisons are to be made between countries, even though in the early stages of the pandemic the statistics were far from being reliable.

Since the number of cases reported per million inhabitants are dependent to a large extent on the capacity of countries to test for the virus, Table 2.2

Table 2.2 COVID-19 cases, deaths and tests, 17 May 2020

Country	Cases absolute numbers	Cases per million	Deaths absolute numbers	Deaths per million	Tests absolute numbers	Tests per million
Belgium	54989	4747	9005	777	663755	57302
Spain	276505	5914	27563	590	3037840	64977
Italy	224760	3717	31763	525	2944859	48698
UK	240161	3540	34466	508	2489563	36696
France	179365	2729	27625	423	1384633	21218
Sweden	29677	2941	3674	364	177500	17589
Netherlands	43870	2561	5670	331	287943	16809
Ireland	24048	4877	1533	311	258808	52488
Luxembourg	3930	6291	104	166	60246	96445
Portugal	28810	2824	1203	118	600061	58828
Germany	176244	2104	8027	96	3147771	37585
Denmark	10858	1875	543	94	444562	76785
Austria	16201	1800	629	70	357393	39710
Romania	16704	868	1094	57	303734	15776
Finland	6286	1135	297	54	143900	25976
Slovenia	1465	705	103	50	68852	33119
Estonia	1770	1334	63	47	68840	51899
Hungary	3509	363	451	47	135173	13985
Czechia	8455	790	296	28	348849	32583
Poland	18257	482	915	24	601394	15888
Croatia	2224	541	95	23	52425	12761
Lithuania	1534	563	55	20	224040	82169
Bulgaria	2211	318	108	16	65574	9429
Greece	2819	270	162	16	126383	12109
Cyprus	914	758	17	14	85301	70715
Malta	546	1237	6	14	49231	111534
Latvia	997	528	19	10	87377	46266
Slovakia	1493	273	28	5	139986	25642
Total	*1378602*		*155514*		*18355993*	

Source: Worldometer (n.d.b).

includes Worldometer's figures for testing. Some countries were testing only patients with severe symptoms that were likely to involve complications, resulting in selection bias (Oke & Heneghan, 2020). By mid-May, Luxembourg was carrying out the largest number of tests per million inhabitants. Greece, Slovakia, Bulgaria, Hungary and Poland were conducting the smallest number. France reported more confirmed cases per million inhabitants than Germany despite carrying out fewer tests. By mid-May, the UK was reporting more cases and deaths than France, and more tests, whereas two weeks earlier the number of tests per million inhabitants in the two countries had been similar. Germany was carrying out testing on a similar scale to the UK but was reporting considerably fewer deaths than might have been expected for its population size (Figure 1.1).

In Italy, where guidelines for classifying COVID-19 fatalities are also known to vary by region, most deaths outside hospitals were not being picked up in the early official statistics. By late April, according to other sources, 'true' deaths due to the virus in the regions most affected by COVID-19 were estimated to be about twice as high as officially reported at national level (Ciminelli & Silvia, 2020).

Belgium and Ireland were reporting similar numbers of cases per million and similar numbers of tests, but different death rates (Table 2.2); they were both including suspected COVID-19-associated deaths based on symptoms. In Belgium, only 17% of the deaths attributed to COVID-19 were confirmed by testing (Laborderie, 2020, p. 4). Cyprus was the last member state to report any cases of infection. By mid-May 2020, with Malta, Luxembourg and Lithuania, Cyprus was one of the countries carrying out the largest number of tests per million inhabitants, suggesting that they were not only testing their whole populations but were also doing so repeatedly.

The relationship between the number of cases and the numbers of deaths per million inhabitants gives an indication of variations in the case fatality rate (the proportion of COVID-19 deaths, compared to the total number of cases diagnosed). On 1 April, Italy, the UK, the Netherlands, Belgium, Spain and France were recording case fatality rates of over 6.5% (Our World in Data, 2020a). The rates in 14 EU member states were 2% or less. Although differences in case fatality rates may be largely explained by discrepancies in data collection practices for the two variables, these findings suggest that the risk of contracting the disease and dying from it are not necessarily directly related and may be attributable to other epidemiological factors (Chapter 5).

COVID-19 deaths in care homes

As the pandemic spread across the EU, and death rates reached over 300 per million inhabitants in Belgium, France, Ireland, Italy, the Netherlands, Spain, Sweden and the UK, attention shifted from deaths in hospitals to those in the community, which had hitherto not always been included in the

Table 2.3 Deaths of care-home residents in selected EU member states, 26 June 2020

Country	Care-home residents' deaths as % of all COVID-19 deaths	COVID-19 deaths as % of all care-home residents	Confirmed/probable COVID-19 deaths
Austria	34	0.3	Confirmed
Belgium	64/50*	4.9	Confirmed & probable
Denmark	35	0.5	Confirmed
Finland	45	nd	Confirmed
France	49/35*	2.4	Confirmed & probable
Germany	39	0.4	Confirmed
Hungary	24	0.2	Confirmed
Ireland	63	3.2	Confirmed & probable
Italy	40*	3.1	Confirmed & probable
Portugal	40	nd	nd
Slovenia	29/52*	0.5	Confirmed
Spain	34(34)	6.1	Confirmed (probable)
Sweden	47	2.8	Confirmed & probable
England & Wales	41/30*	3.4	Confirmed & probable
Northern Ireland	52/43*	nd	Confirmed & probable
Scotland	44/47*	nd	Confirmed & probable

Source: Comas-Herrera et al. (2020, tables 1 and 2).
* Deaths in care homes

statistics. The LSE Care Policy and Evaluation Centre (CPEC) noted the difficulties in making international comparisons of COVID-19-associated deaths for care-homes residents owing to differences in testing capacity, recording practices and policy, all of which were evolving over time, and to the lack of reliable data for many of the countries they were studying. From the data that they were able to assemble, the team identified three approaches to quantifying COVID-19 deaths: people who test positive (before or after death), people suspected of having COVID-19 (based on symptoms) and excess deaths, resulting in under- and over-estimations (Table 2.3).

CPEC postulated a relationship between the percentage of COVID-19-related deaths among care-home residents and the total number of deaths in the whole population. This observation was not borne out when deaths among care-home residents are considered as a proportion of all COVID-19 deaths per million inhabitants: Austria, Denmark, Finland, Hungary and Slovenia consistently reported similar relatively low death rates per million inhabitants overall, but varying percentages for care-home deaths in relation to all COVID-19 deaths. The relatively low figure for Hungary would seem to be attributable to the small proportion (3%) of older people living in care homes (Comas-Herrera et al., 2020).

Germany included confirmed deaths in all communal establishments extending to community facilities for asylum seekers, homeless shelters and prisons. Information on the care setting was missing in 37% of reported cases. CPEC estimated that care-home residents represented a smaller share of all deaths in Germany compared to other countries with similar total numbers of deaths. In Sweden, which also reported only confirmed deaths, 14% of all COVID-19 positive confirmed cases were occurring among care-home residents. By 12 May 2020, cases of infection had been reported in all care homes in the Stockholm region. Two days later, 48.9% of all deaths in Sweden, where COVID-19 was mentioned on the death certificate, were of care-home residents. The similarly high figures for Belgium and Ireland, which both counted confirmed and probable cases, do not reflect the large difference in their overall numbers of deaths per million population. France began including deaths in care homes in its returns on 4 April, but also provided separate counts for the number of care-home residents who died in hospital.

In France, Italy, Spain and the UK, regional variations could be observed. CPEC data for Italy were based on a survey representing just over 10% of the country's care homes. By early May, 13% of care-home deaths were reported in Lombardy compared to 7% in Veneto. In Spain, some regions differentiated between deaths of people diagnosed with COVID-19 and those with symptoms who had not been diagnosed, while other regions did not make that distinction. In the UK, statistics for deaths in different settings were broken down by nation (Table 2.3).

When COVID-19 deaths are considered in relation to all care-home residents in the countries for which data are available, Germany, Denmark, Slovenia and Austria, which displayed the lowest rates, were clearly distinguished from the countries with the highest rates: Spain, Belgium, the UK, Ireland, Italy, Sweden and France. The fact that the first grouping of countries did not include probable cases only partially explains the differences between the two groupings.

Tracking excess mortality

The CPEC team were also interested in excess deaths, but the data they assembled did not enable them to pursue this aspect in their study. Other researchers have also been hampered by the limited information available, since few countries systematically collect comparable longitudinal data, and none of the institutions monitoring excess mortality cover all EU member states. Table 2.4 displays Z-scores from EuroMOMO (2020b) for the weeks when death rates peaked in each of the countries they studied, and at week 25 when the spike of the pandemic had passed. For their country peak weeks, Spain and England recorded the highest scores, followed by Belgium, France and the Netherlands. They were all countries reporting high numbers of deaths at 1 April (Table 2.1). Greece, Hungary, Estonia and Denmark displayed very low Z-scores in line with their much lower numbers of deaths.

By week 25, the EuroMOMO (2020b) network noted in its weekly bulletin that, in most countries, levels had returned to normal or were even

Table 2.4 Z-scores for excess mortality, selected EU member states, by ages and peak weeks

Country	Country peak week	Z-score at peak week	Z-score week 25	Z-score aged 65+	Z-scores aged 75+	Older age peak week
Austria	14	3.51	−0.67	−0.67	4.49	14
Belgium	15	24.14	4.77	4.80	20.84	15
Denmark	15	1.89	−1.04	−1.19	2.91	14
Estonia	17	1.31	0.05	−0.44	1.16	19
Finland	15	2.50	−1.12	−0.99	4.10	16
France	14	23.79	−9.08	−7.74	20.77	14
Berlin	15	1.50	−0.98	−1.04	2.31	14
Greece	20	1.24	0.41	0.56	3.02	5
Hungary	15	1.37	−1.44	−1.75	1.87	12
Ireland	15	9.37	−2.24	−2.92	7.34	15
Italy	14	16.79	−1.72	−1.75	13.74	13
Luxembourg	15	3.00	0.59	0.48	5.55	15
Malta	16	2.88	0.96	0.81	3.84	16
Netherlands	14	21.74	0.47	0.46	15.69	14
Portugal	14	5.40	−0.44	−0.38	4.39	15
Spain	14	43.57	3.63	3.32	44.44	13
Sweden	15	12.93	2.32	2.15	10.82	16
England	15	40.76	0.08	0.07	29.42	15
N Ireland	15	9.15	−3.58	−3.08	5.91	17
Scotland	15	15.92	0.04	0.50	12.08	16
Wales	15	18.81	−6.33	−6.12	14.36	15

Source: EuroMOMO (2020b).

lower than in previous years. A few countries, Belgium and Spain, were still seeing some excess mortality. The mortality data in Spain had been corrected upwards, to take account of under-notification of deaths in the civil registers during the early phase of the COVID-19 pandemic. The Z-scores for EuroMOMO also showed that excess mortality for the older age groups had peaked, in most cases at the same time as it spiked for all age groups. Austria and Greece peaked much earlier for the older age groups, and Estonia somewhat later. By week 25 (mid-June), most countries were recording very low, if not negative, excess death rates among older age groups. Only Belgium, Spain and Sweden were still displaying Z-scores greater than 2. EuroMOMO noted, however, that excess mortality was also being observed in the 45−64 and 15−44 age groups.

Since EuroMOMO provides Z-score for Berlin and the nations in the UK, Table 2.4 uses information prepared by two data journalists for the BBC to set Germany and the UK in relation to indicators for excess mortality in nine of the countries featured in Table 2.5 (Dale & Stylianou, 2020). Their animated guide plots excess mortality that may have been directly or indirectly caused by COVID-19 averaged over several weeks and encompassing people who would have been expected to die around that time if the pandemic had not occurred. Their analysis suggests that Spain, the UK,

Table 2.5 Excess deaths in selected EU member states, 2 March–5 June 2020

Country	Duration of pandemic	Excess deaths	% above expected average
Austria	16 March–10 May	1300	11
Belgium	9 March–17 May	8100	37
Denmark	16 March–10May	400	4
France	2 March–10 May	28400	25
Germany	9 March–10 May	7100	4
Italy	24 February–26 Apr	42900	40
Netherlands	9 March–24 May	9600	30
Portugal	16 March–17 May	2800	15
Spain	2 March–17 May	42900	50
Sweden	9 March–17 May	4200	24
UK	7 March–5 June	64500	43

Source: Dale & Stylianou (2020).

Italy and Belgium were well above the expected average, while Denmark, Germany and Austria were well below.

Whatever measurement system is used, England records relatively high scores, well about those for the other nations in the UK. Aron & Muellbauer (2020) attribute this finding, among others, to high average infection rates in preceding weeks due to the London-centric location of the spread of the pandemic.

Setting COVID-19 deaths in relation to socio-demographic and public health indicators

Absolute numbers of deaths are relevant for analysts tracking the progression of the pandemic over time in individual countries. When EU member states are being compared, the absolute numbers of deaths reported in the headlines misrepresent the situation because they do not take account of relative population size. Nor are they found to match closely estimates based on the other socio-demographic characteristics reviewed in Chapter 1.

The patterning displayed in Figure 1.9 is suggestive of how a combination of factors may help to explain the positioning of different member states in Table 2.2. The position of countries recording the highest absolute numbers of deaths (the UK, Italy, France, Spain, Belgium, Germany, the Netherlands, Sweden and Ireland) on 17 May 2020 changes when the numbers are considered in relation to population size, density and old-age dependency (Figure 1.1). France, the UK, Italy and Spain, with their relatively large population sizes remain among the countries recording the highest numbers of deaths per million inhabitants, as do the Netherlands given their population size and density. Germany records a much smaller number of deaths in absolute and relative terms than might have been expected for its population size (Hamann, 2020). Despite its similarity to the Netherlands in terms of population size and density, Belgium emerges as an outlier owing to its very large number of COVID-19 deaths.

Other clusters of countries can be identified based on their demographic characteristics: Cyprus, Malta and Luxembourg for their small population size and high density; Croatia, Estonia, Latvia, Lithuania, Slovakia and Slovenia for small population size but relatively low density; or Denmark, Finland, Ireland and Sweden for their small population size and relatively low density. In most cases, these countries report relatively low numbers of COVID-19 deaths, but some of the largest numbers of tests. Ireland and Sweden are noteworthy for their relatively high numbers of deaths in relation to their demographic characteristics, and Greece for its low numbers of cases, deaths and tests, given its demographic profile.

When demographic statistics are examined in conjunction with health indicators, different patterns emerge in relation to COVID-19 cases. Countries that devote a relatively large proportion of their GDP and per capita expenditure to healthcare provision and protection, whether funded by taxation or insurance, might be expected to report lower case fatality rates. To what extent this commitment to healthcare mitigates, or the lack of it exacerbates, the effects of other factors is variable, as illustrated by France, Germany, Sweden and the UK, on the one hand, and Estonia, Romania and Slovenia, on the other hand.

The analysis in this chapter of some of the many factors contributing to variations in death rates, particularly excess mortality (Tallack et al., 2020), highlights major differences not only between countries but also within them between regions and localities. This observation illustrates the complexity of the situation across the EU and the importance of identifying similarities and differences in background factors when making comparisons of COVID-19 cases and deaths.

3 Tracking and comparing government responses to COVID-19

This chapter reviews the measures taken by governments to contain the spread of the virus, and the exit strategies they adopted to ease lockdown. Difficulties were encountered in collating precise, reliable and consistent data about the timing of the onset of COVID-19 and its peaks, the speed and intensity with which measures were implemented, and the strictness of their application. Some EU member states made recommendations and issued advice, others introduced restrictive measures progressively, while yet others declared an emergency and imposed a draconian lockdown with penalties for non-compliance. Various combinations of measures were introduced covering the banning of public events, social gatherings, internal and external travel, school and shop closures, and social distancing. Research institutions developed models for assessing the effectiveness of different measures in containing the disease, including a COVID-19 stringency index of government responses and lockdown rollback checklist. The analysis shows how, in many countries, the introduction of restrictive measures was less controversial than decisions about lifting or easing lockdown, as governments, ministers of finance and health grappled with conflicting interests, pressures and advice.

Introducing lockdown

The respective public health competences of EU institutions and member states are clearly laid down in treaties. Public health is an area of policy, like social protection, where national governments retain responsibility for formulating and implementing national-level policy. In their capacity as members of the European Council, the EU's main decision-making body, heads of state or government are involved in determining EU as well as national-level policy. EU institutions are charged with ensuring a high level of human health protection, with coordinating action between member states and cooperating with them to prevent diseases and combat cross-border threats to health (Article 129, 1992 Maastricht Treaty), as well as promoting research into the causes and transmission of 'major health scourges'.

The World Health Organisation (WHO, 2020d) recognised Europe as the epicentre of the pandemic on 13 March 2020. Without waiting for instructions from EU institutions, and without having available reliable scientific evidence with which to assess their likely impact, national and local governments exercised their responsibility by introducing a combination of measures to contain or suppress the spread of the disease among their populations (COVID–DEM Infohub, 2020; Politico EU, 2020b). This section reviews the mix of government interventions and the pace at which they were implemented.

EU and national restrictions on travel and public events

Operating within its mandate for ensuring coordinated action, on 11 March 2020, the European Commission president, Ursula von der Leyen, proposed the shutdown of external borders in both directions to limit the spread of the COVID-19 outbreak. The European Council endorsed the proposal the following day. By then, almost all EU member states had imposed restrictions on travel to and from Italy. A few days later, the European Commission (2020, 16 March) issued a Communication recommending temporary restrictions (for 30 days in the first instance) on non-essential travel. These restrictions were designed to stem the number of imported COVID-19 cases, thereby easing pressures on national healthcare systems while also preventing the spread of the virus from the EU to other countries.

Although, under EU law, the Commission did not have the power to enforce restrictions within member states, it stressed that, to be effective, any coordinating action recommended needed to be applied to all the EU's external borders. Exemptions to travel restrictions were made for EU nationals, residents and family members returning home, as well as for other categories such as essential workers, frontier workers and haulage transporters. The same Communication specified that the restrictions should include the non-Schengen EU member states, namely Bulgaria, Croatia, Cyprus and Romania. Ireland and the UK were also invited to align with the EU's advice. UK nationals were to be treated in the same way as EU citizens until the end of 2020 when the arrangements for implementing Brexit should have been agreed. According to observers of the European scene, the hope was that closure of the bloc's external borders would convince EU member states to avoid imposing restrictions within the EU on grounds that they would endanger the functioning of the highly integrated Single Market (Bayer & Cokeleare, 2020).

By mid-March 2020, the 22 EU Schengen countries (Table 4.1) individually initiated travel bans and closed their borders to stem the spread of the virus, thereby flouting the EU's freedom of movement principle (Box 3.1). In a second Communication concerning the implementation of restrictions on non-essential travel, the European Commission (2020, 30 March) recommended limiting the number of border crossing points for categories of travellers allowed to enter the Schengen area to facilitate document checks and other controls. Without further comment, the Commission noted that several countries had decided to put everyone entering their country, including their own citizens, into quarantine for 14 days. Austria had already placed certain towns under full quarantine. Third countries were reciprocating by quarantining travellers from EU member states: Hong Kong, for example, had decided to quarantine all visitors from Italy and affected parts of France and Germany for two weeks from 13 March.

Box 3.1 Closure of national borders

Governments in Czechia, Denmark, Greece, Hungary, Latvia, Lithuania, Poland and Slovakia completely closed internal borders. Belgium, Germany, Slovenia and Sweden closed their borders for non-essential travel. Finland temporarily banned travel abroad. Italy kept its borders open but restricted entry from neighbouring countries, and Spain stopped all flights to and from Italy. The Netherlands limited entry for non-EU citizens, while Portugal constrained movement from Spain. Austria and Estonia imposed restrictions and introduced health screening at borders, whereas France, Luxembourg and Malta kept their borders open. Reactions in the non-Schengen countries were equally diverse: Cyprus closed its borders, Bulgaria and Croatia stopped international flights. Romania stopped travel to France, Germany, Italy and Spain, whereas Ireland and the UK kept their borders open (Bayer & Cokeleare, 2020; Hantrais 2020a; Hirsch, 2020).

In addition to external movement, member states unilaterally imposed restrictions on internal movement, as they were entitled to do under EU law. The measures implemented included confinement or self-isolation for vulnerable categories, their shielders and anyone infected by the virus. Regional variations operated within countries at the discretion of local authorities (Bulgaria, France, Germany, Italy and the UK). Public transport services were curtailed and/or limited to key workers. All but essential travel by car was outlawed or discouraged in most countries. Exceptions were generally made to restrictions on internal movement for shopping, banking, medical appointments or the collection of medicines, with fines for non-compliance.

The European Commission did not issue guidance on the banning of public events and gatherings. As the number of deaths associated with the virus grew exponentially, individual member states introduced bans on different group activities and limited the size of public gatherings (Box 3.2). Most sporting events and activities were cancelled *sine die* across the EU. Theatres, cinemas, concert halls, opera houses, libraries and museums were closed, and religious and social ceremonies, including attendance at weddings and funerals, were banned within days of reporting the first cases (Henley, 2020; Hirsch, 2020).

Box 3.2 Bans on public events and gatherings

Most countries allowed physical exercise or walking pets in the open air, but not in groups or with a non-household member. In many cases, all face-to-face contact was limited to immediate family members except in essential public services. In the UK, outside exercise was allowed only once a day for an hour. France and Italy permitted only walking alone and close to home (within one kilometre in France). Both countries introduced self-certification, as did Greece and Romania. Forms with name, date, time and reason for authorised travel had to be completed by anyone leaving their home. In Hungary, anyone in compulsory home quarantine was obliged to post a sign from the authorities ('a red card') on their door to warn others that a potentially infected person inside was under disease control observation by the police (Kovács, 2020).

Parks and beaches were closed. Belgium did not allow sitting in parks, and Bulgaria banned jogging or walking. Spain did not allow parents to take children out for shopping unless it was impossible to leave them at home alone. France did not allow cycling for sport. Poland banned young people under the age of 13 from leaving their homes unattended; access to all public green spaces and beaches was prohibited as well as the use of city bikes (Jaraczewski, 2020; Republic of Poland, 2020), while in many countries, the UK for example, cycling became a popular form of exercise and a highly recommended mode of travel.

Some countries set different limits for indoor and outdoor events, as awareness grew that the risk of transmission was greater in enclosed spaces. For example, Austria, Hungary, Ireland and Slovenia banned outdoor gatherings of more than 500 people and indoor events of more than 100, Portugal allowed 1,000 inside and 5,000 outside, and Romania 100 and 1,000 respectively.

Belgium's prime minister, Sophie Wilmès, recommended that indoor events with more than 1,000 people be postponed. Poland banned all mass events, while the ban in Slovenia operated for gatherings of more than 1,000 people. Berlin became the seventh of Germany's 16 states to ban gatherings of 1,000 people or more, illustrating the importance of regional differentiation in timing and of variations within countries that delegated decision-making powers. Czechia and Romania banned all events involving more than 100 people, and Ireland cancelled St Patrick's Day parades on 17 March. France initially banned all gatherings of more than 5,000 people but went ahead with the first round of municipal elections on 15 March 2020. The second round, which was due to be held a week later, was postponed until 28 June. In the UK, mass gatherings were banned from 20 March, although many organisations had already decided to cancel public events, including sports fixtures and concerts well ahead of any official ban.

Spain closed the lower house of parliament for at least a week after one MP tested positive. In the UK, parliament and courts began working remotely, as did courts in Romania for example. Cyprus, Italy and Malta suspended the operation of their courts, Greece suspended trials in court. Courts were partially closed in Denmark. Estonia banned public hearings. Courts were closed in Hungary and Poland, and they were not fully functioning in Bulgaria (COVID–DEM Infohub, 2020).

Closure of educational institutions, shops, offices and the hospitality industry

During the month of March, in line with bans on public events and gatherings, most EU member states closed down shops, factories, offices, schools and the hospitality industry, but allowed banks and retail outlets producing and/or selling groceries and other essential goods such as medical supplies to remain open, provided they observed precautionary measures (Box 3.3).

Box 3.3 Closure of workplaces and schools

Denmark and Sweden did not introduce formal closures of workplaces and schools, and a few governments – Croatia, Estonia, Germany, Hungary, Luxembourg, Slovakia – announced only partial closures (Hirsch, 2020). Workers able to do so were encouraged, advised or instructed to work from home, using technological solutions to stay connected. Provision for online shopping and home deliveries expanded rapidly to meet the demand. The hospitality industry (cafés, restaurants, hotels, tourism) were among the industries hardest hit by lockdown; most of their employees were either furloughed or made redundant, but some outlets continued to operate by providing takeaway services and home deliveries, and some suppliers transferred their product sales to retail outlets.

In Italy, the European country first affected by the pandemic, nurseries and schools closed on the 5 March 2020. This decision was soon followed by Greece, Czechia and Romania. Most European education systems had temporarily closed their institutions by 16 March 2020. In some countries – Belgium, Italy, the Netherlands, France and the UK – nurseries and schools remained open for children whose parents were key workers, and to support vulnerable children. Sweden kept

day-care centres and primary schools open without any major adjust-
ments to class size, lunch policies, or recess rules. Individual schools
opted to close temporarily when an outbreak of the virus occurred
(Vogel, 2020).

In the UK, which was the last country to announce formal closure,
it was estimated that by 20–23 March, only about 10% of children in
England were still attending school. The government issued guidance
on 19 March to ensure that, during the COVID-19 outbreak, children
who were eligible for benefits-related free school meals would receive
meals or food vouchers while they were not attending school (UK
Government Department for Education, 2020).

Nursery and school closures proved to be controversial. Although scientific evidence confirmed that young children were less likely than older
people to contract the disease and die from it, scientists, educationalists and
parents were divided about the long-term impact on children's physical and
mental health, and risks to the development of their social skills and com-
petencies. Eurydice (2020), a European network of 43 national units based
in the 38 countries operating the Erasmus+ programme, assessed the process and impact of school closures in early April. On the positive side, they
observed how teaching had moved online for those equipped to deliver and
receive remote learning packages. Learning support was being provided using books and materials taken from schools; e-learning platforms enabled
teachers and pupils to work and interact together, assisted by national tele-
vision programmes and/or lessons on social media platforms.

Eurydice recognised, however, that school closure put new pressures on
parents as well as producing negative educational impacts. The network
raised questions concerning grading and assessment of progress, as well as
the organisation of final exams or national tests. Some parents were unable
to support their children's learning effectively; economically and socially
disadvantaged pupils were found to be less likely to have access to learning
materials, including online platforms, and to receive support, thereby intensifying existing educational inequalities.

Although universities, including in Sweden, stopped providing lectures
and other face-to-face classes, often on their own initiative, they did not all
'close for business'. Provision was made for delivering lectures, panel discussions and debates online, and innovative methods were found for tutoring
and assessment, using Zoom and webinars.

Rules on physical distancing

Governments across the EU introduced some form of physical distancing
and self-isolation of infected and vulnerable people to contain transmission

of the virus and shield the categories of the population most at risk, especially older people with underlying health conditions. Following the review of social distancing measures in their broader sense, this section focusses on the narrower meaning of the term referring to the physical or spatial distance to be observed between people in situations where social interaction and contact are necessary and allowed, whether it be in shops, offices, public transport or open spaces (Box 3.4). As the outbreak gained pandemic proportions, physical distancing rules were widely and readily accepted by most people as the price to pay for avoiding complete shutdowns of whole societies. In Sweden, the country most resistant to state interventions, citizens were expected to take individual responsibility for physical distancing, in return for which the government would keep most of society functioning (Anderson, 2020).

Box 3.4 Guidance on physical distancing

On 23 March 2020, the European Centre for Disease Prevention and Control (ECDC), an EU agency based in Sweden, issued an update on social distancing. ECDC (2020a, pp. 1, 3) described social distancing as 'an action taken to minimise contact with other individuals … aimed at reducing disease transmission and thereby also reducing pressure on health services'. ECDC cautioned that, if it is to be effective over an extended period, social distancing should not prevent 'social contact – from a distance – with friends, family and colleagues'. Internet-based communications were therefore recommended as 'a key tool for ensuring a successful social distancing strategy'.

The available scientific evidence was inconclusive about the optimal distance that needed to be observed to curb the spread of the virus, resulting in different practices being observed. A systematic review published in the *Lancet* (Chu et al., 2020, p. 1974) suggested that: 'From a policy and public health perspective, current policies of at least 1 m physical distancing seem to be strongly associated with a large protective effect, and distances of 2 m could be more effective'. The findings from their review observed that a physical distance of one meter in both healthcare and community settings 'is strongly associated with protection against the virus, but that distances up to two meters might be more effective' (Chu et al., 2020, p. 1984). This evidence has since been widely used to support community physical distancing guidelines and to demonstrate the feasibility of risk reduction by physical distancing.

Bischoff (2020), a scientist at the Wake Forest School of Medicine in North Carolina, argued that maximum transmission of the virus, particularly indoors and after prolonged exposure, took place at one meter. Thereafter, as the size of airborne droplets decreased, the likelihood of transmission diminished, suggesting that different distances could be observed outdoors and indoors.

WHO (n.d.a) recommended physical distancing of 'at least 1 metre'. As with other measures, physical distancing was implemented differentially both within and between member states based on each government's preferred scientific advice and political priorities. Bulgaria, France and Italy adopted 1 meter, whereas Belgium, Germany and the Netherlands observed 1.5 meters, and Austria, Spain and the UK chose 2 meters. In guidelines issued on 21 May, the European Union Aviation Safety Agency and ECDC (EASA/ECDC, 2020) settled on 1.5 meter for airlines, where operationally feasible, to ensure uniformity across the EU.

As governments encouraged those who could not work at home to return to their workplaces, they relied on physical distancing in public spaces to continue to slow the spread of the virus. The numbers of passengers in public transport were to be limited to ensure physical distancing, and airlines announced that they would be leaving empty seats and rows to limit physical contact. Floor markers and screens were introduced in supermarkets, for queuing and for small gatherings in public spaces. Desks and workstations in schools and offices were kept apart in 'bubbles'. In the few countries where attendance at mass gatherings was not prohibited, measures were implemented to limit physical contact by keeping seats empty, as practised, for example, in cinemas in Bulgaria.

Although most member states imposed strict physical distancing rules within their own borders, these measures were not always applied to nationals from other countries. For example, seasonal workers from Bulgaria, Romania and Poland travelled on chartered flights to other EU member states to harvest crops, as they had done in previous years. On 2 April, Germany lifted its ban on seasonal farm workers entering the country, announcing that farms could bring in 80,000 seasonal labourers in April and May. Workers from Romania complained that hygiene and social distancing rules were not being respected, and that living conditions were unsafe (Neagu, 2020; Poenaru & Rogozanu, 2020). Other countries reported similar abuses of physical distancing rules as they struggled to prevent harvests being lost in the absence of local workers (Bodeux & Gnes, 2020), or became aware of poor working conditions in food processing plants (Foote, 2020).

Rules on the wearing of face coverings

In the absence of consistent evidence about the wearing of face coverings, member states wavered in their approach: initially the wearing of face masks and/or gloves was made mandatory in public places in Austria, Bulgaria, Czechia, France, Germany, Lithuania, Poland and Slovakia. It was not considered necessary or advisable in Ireland, Sweden and the UK when other interventions were being implemented. Gradually consensus grew that the effectiveness of face coverings outside clinical settings depended on a societal approach being adopted based on the precautionary principle (Box 3.5). Other elementary measures, for example, hand hygiene, were widely recommended in addition to physical distancing and use of face masks.

Box 3.5 Guidance on face coverings

Advice on the wearing of face masks and other face coverings was inconsistent. In June 2020, WHO updated its strategy on masks in the context of COVID-19, cautiously observing that:

> Non-medical, fabric masks are being used by many people in public areas, but there has been limited evidence on their effectiveness and WHO does not recommend their widespread use among the public for control of COVID-19. However, for areas of widespread transmission, with limited capacity for implementing control measures and especially in settings where physical distancing of at least 1 metre is not possible – such as on public transport, in shops or in other confined or crowded environments – WHO advises governments to encourage the general public to use non-medical fabric masks.
>
> (WHO, 2020b)

In the same document, WHO described the intention behind face coverings as two-fold: 'preventing the wearer transmitting infection to others (source control) or to offer protection to the wearer against infection (prevention)'. WHO recommended that people aged over 60, or anyone of any age with an underlying health condition or their carers should wear a medical-grade mask in public settings.

At EU level, ECDC (2020d) was also cautious, stating:

> It should be emphasised that use of face masks in the community should be considered **only as a complementary measure** and not as a replacement of the core preventive measures that are recommended to reduce community transmission including physical distancing, staying home when ill, teleworking if possible, respiratory etiquette, meticulous hand hygiene and avoiding touching the face, nose, eyes and mouth.
>
> (ECDC, 2020d, p. 3, original emphasis)

Promotion of hand hygiene

Even before unprecedented social distancing interventions became mandatory, a long-established public health, and largely uncontroversial, measure
was being promulgated by international and national institutions. Hand
hygiene had proven to be effective in preventing the spread of diseases in
hospitals as early as the mid-1800s. After widespread testing in hospitals
around the world, WHO (2009) adopted a hand hygiene improvement strategy for translating its recommendations into practice. Within the context
of their Year of the Nurse and Midwife, WHO (2020c) designated 5 May
2020 as Hand Hygiene Day to be celebrated with 'clapping for nurses and
midwives at noon on 5 May to thank and recognize their critical role in
delivering clean care'.

WHO (2020a) portrayed hand hygiene as 'the most effective single measure to reduce the spread of infections'. For EU member states, hand washing
with soap and water offered a seemingly simple but effective action that was
quickly adopted by policymakers and the public at large[1].

The promotion of hand washing created an unprecedented demand for
hand sanitisers, resulting in panic buying, inflated prices and shortages, and
bans on exports within and outside the EU of sanitisers and other personal
protective equipment (PPE). Although PPE was mandatory for frontline
workers, many countries struggled to meet the demand. On 3 March 2020,
the French government took control of production of personal protective
equipment (PPE), requisitioning face masks and capping the price of sanitis-
ing gel. Germany followed with an export ban on PPE, while Italy, Czechia
and Poland resorted to imports from Russia and China (Braw, 2020; Macek,
2020).

National approaches to lockdown

Amidst conflicting scientific evidence and advice from international institutions, national governments had to decide whether, when and how to intervene to control the spread of the COVID-19 pandemic, to relieve pressure
on their health services and limit damage to their economies. This section
examines the introduction and easing of lockdown measures across EU
member states.

Timing of lockdown

All EU member states progressively introduced protective and preventative measures in different combinations and sequences, at different times,
in different localities and with different degrees of severity, making it difficult to determine the extent and timing of lockdown, and complicating
analysis of its possible effects on both social and economic life. A chart
produced by the BBC (2020) analysing the severity of restrictions on internal
movement in European countries distinguished between nationalised and

localised recommendations and lockdown. The chart shows how most countries introduced national lockdown without first practising local lockdown. Austria, Bulgaria, Germany, Greece and Italy initially introduced localised lockdown before issuing national instructions. Hungary, Latvia and Sweden made only national recommendations, while Finland and Malta implemented localised measures after first issuing national recommendations.

Politico EU (Hirsch, 2020) tabulated the number of days between the date when the first deaths were recorded and the date of implementation of each measure in 12 member states. The COVID–DEM Infohub (2020) provided details about the timing and legislative frameworks of emergency measures across EU member states (Chapter 4). Table 3.1 draws together information from these different sources to provide an indication of the relationship between the timing of the third COVID-19 death (as reported in Table 2.1) and the dates when states of emergency (indicated in bold) or national

Table 3.1 Days between third deaths and lockdown, by dates

Country	Date of 3rd death	Official lockdown date	Days 3rd death to lockdown
Austria	17 March	15 March	−2
Belgium	12 March	27 March	15
Bulgaria	19 March	**23 March**	4
Croatia	26 March	19 March	−7
Cyprus	25 March	*24 March	−1
Czechia	25 March	**12 March**	−13
Denmark	16 March	*19 March	3
Estonia	30 March	**12 March**	−18
Finland	28 March	**16 March**	−12
France	3 March	16/**23 March**	13/20
Germany	12 March	25 March	13
Greece	15 March	*24 March	9
Hungary	21 March	30 March	9
Ireland	15 March	*27 March	12
Italy	25 February	**31 January**	−25
Latvia	11 April	**12 March**	−30
Lithuania	25 March	26 February	−28
Luxembourg	19 March	**16 March**	−3
Malta	11 April	12 March	−30
Netherlands	9 March	17 March	8
Poland	15 March	2/**31 March**	−13/16
Portugal	20 March	12 March	−8
Romania	22 March	9/**16 March**	−13/−6
Slovakia	15 April	**19/25 March**	−26/−21
Slovenia	23 April	12 March	−42
Spain	6 March	14 March	8
Sweden	16 March	4 April	19
UK	9 March	23 March	14

Sources: BBC (2020): national lockdown dates; COVID–DEM Infohub (2020): official lockdown dates; Politico EU (n.d.b): third deaths.
Bold: States of emergency
* National lockdowns

lockdown was announced. The figures in the table should be treated with caution since measures were rarely introduced simultaneously and across whole countries, and states of emergency were sometimes declared or implemented retroactively.

When the relationship between the dates for the first three deaths and national lockdown are considered, the figures reveal further differences between countries. The first lockdown was introduced on 12 March in five countries. In 16 countries, lockdown preceded the third death. Slovenia acted well ahead of an anticipated rising death toll, as did Malta, Lithuania, Slovakia, Italy and Latvia. Of these, Slovakia, Italy and Latvia all declared a state of emergency, signalling that they were intending to impose stringent and timely measures to deal with the crisis. Estonia, Czechia, Finland and Luxembourg also declared a state of emergency before reporting their third COVID-19 death. Bulgaria and Romania made their declaration within a few days of the third death. They were among the countries that did not introduce a state of emergency. Denmark implemented national lockdown within a few days of the third death. Belgium, France, Germany, Ireland, Sweden and the UK took more than 10 days before introducing centralised nationwide lockdown, often resulting in criticism of politicians for the delay.

The Imperial College COVID-19 Response Team attempted to assess whether changes in death rates in March 2020 might be attributable to policy measures (Flaxman et al., 2020). The study included 11 EU member states. The team calculated backwards from the deaths observed over time to estimate transmission that occurred several weeks earlier, taking account of the time lag between infection and death. One of their key assumptions was that each intervention (school closures, bans on public events, social distancing, lockdown decrees) had the same effect across countries and over time. They estimated that major non-pharmaceutical interventions had a substantial impact on the time-varying infection rates in countries where there had been time to observe intervention effects on trends in deaths (Italy and Spain) (Flaxman et al., 2020, p. 13). They acknowledged, however, that, due to the implementation of interventions in rapid succession in many countries, the available data did not suffice to determine the size of the individual effect of each intervention. Despite their dubious assumptions and caveats, their timeline for interventions is useful since it confirms that, in the countries studied, official lockdown often followed, rather than preceded, the introduction of individual measures.

Preparing for lockdown exit

On 15 April 2020, ministers of health for EU27 member states held a video conference to take stock of the current situation and measures implemented in response to the spread of COVID-19 in the EU (European Council, 2020b). They exchanged views on a common exit strategy for de-escalation of containment measures. Their discussions focussed on working together towards a common EU exit strategy, aimed at improving coordination across the EU, identifying the most appropriate time for relaxing the measures and providing clear information and guidance to the public.

The next day, the Commission produced a European Roadmap towards lifting COVID-19 containment measures. In presenting the Roadmap, the Commission reiterated the widespread concerns expressed by EU member states, claiming that

> ...restrictive measures have been necessary to slow down the spread of the virus and have already saved tens of thousands of lives. But they come at a high social and economic cost. They put a strain on mental health and force citizens to radically change their day-to-day lives. They have created huge shocks to the economy and seriously impacted the functioning of the Single Market, in that whole sectors are closed down, connectivity is significantly limited and international supply chains and people's freedom of movement have been severely disrupted. This has triggered the need for public intervention to counterbalance the socio-economic impact, both at EU and Member State levels.
>
> (European Commission, 2020, 16 April, p. 2)

The Commission recognised that the way back to normality would be long, and that de-escalation from COVID-19 required proportionate measures that could be revised as knowledge of the virus and the disease evolved. Following ECDC (2020b) guidance issued earlier in the month, the Roadmap was based on three key criteria, principles or pre-conditions for easing lockdown: epidemiological criteria showing that the spread of the disease had significantly decreased; sufficient health system capacity, for example, taking into account the occupation rate for intensive care units, the availability of healthcare workers and medical material; appropriate monitoring capacity, including large-scale testing capacity to detect and isolate infected individuals rapidly, as well as tracking and tracing capacity. Arguably, the Commission was acting in accordance with its limited public health mandate by stressing the need for a coordinated but gradual exit strategy, allowing for local and national specificities, and in consultation with heads of state or government.

As the full social and economic impacts of the pandemic became apparent, and public opinion and confidence in government shifted (see Chapter 4), member states faced even greater challenges than when lockdown was being introduced. National governments continued to exercise their responsibility by taking and implementing decisions concerning public health policies and opening up their economies as and when they considered that the time was right. It is therefore difficult to identify precise dates when restrictions were lifted across a range of measures and to estimate the length of time that countries were under full lockdown. Both entry and exit were progressive and were influenced by a variety of medical and non-medical factors.

Assessing readiness for lockdown exit

Understanding how best to control the spread of virus is dependent on being able to assess the effectiveness of the measures introduced to contain it and to mitigate its effects. ECDC (2020c) continued to monitor and report on the epidemiological situation and to make risk assessments as the prevalence of the pandemic lessened. Meanwhile, research teams in Europe were developing datasets that could be used to monitor and document the impact of lockdown measures and to assess the readiness of member states to exit lockdown (Box 3.6).

Box 3.6 Monitoring COVID-19 lockdown measures

Drawing on a variety of sources, the Oxford Blavatnik School (n.d.a) created the Oxford COVID-19 government response tracker to document government responses in countries worldwide. The tracker, which covered all EU member states, was designed to enable researchers, policymakers and citizens to review, analyse and compare government responses to the pandemic in selected countries. The aim was to monitor how the spread of the disease evolved over time as policy measures took effect.

Countries at an early stage of the outbreak were invited to use the stringency index (Oxford Blavatnik School, n.d.b) to observe how other countries that were already at a later stage (for example Italy) had responded to the pandemic The Oxford COVID-19 stringency index provides composite scores for a series of 17 indicators assessing the strictness of government responses over several months: eight of their policy indicators (C1-C8) record information on containment and closure policies, such as school closures and restrictions on movement; four of the indicators (E1-E4) record economic policies, such as income support to citizens or provision of foreign aid; and five indicators (H1-H5) record health system policies such as the COVID-19 testing regimes or emergency investments in healthcare.

The Oxford COVID-19 government response tracker team also produced a lockdown rollback checklist showing which countries came near to meeting four of the WHO's six recommendations for relaxing physical distancing measures: transmission under control; health system capacity; outbreak risks in high-vulnerability settings minimised; preventive measures in workplaces; managed risk of transmission; and prevention strategies in place (Petherick et al., 2020). Their composite indicator (OxCGRT) covered cases controlled, test, trace and isolate, manage imported cases and community understanding in all EU member states except Malta, Latvia and Lithuania. While the checklist could not be used to determine with certainty how ready countries were to leave lockdown, it offered a rough indication across member states on a scale from 0.0 to 0.9 (Hale et al., 2020).

A team of scientists at the Unit of Public Health and Epidemiology in Vienna (Desvars-Larrive et al., 2020) developed a structured open dataset of government interventions in response to COVID-19. Their algorithms were designed to analyse how, during the COVID-19 pandemic, governments enforced a broad spectrum of intervention measures, under rapidly changing, unprecedented circumstances. The team set out to assess community mitigation strategies aimed at preventing the introduction of infectious diseases (preparedness and readiness measures), containing their spread and reducing the burden on health systems (control measures). They included records for 13 EU member states: Austria, Belgium, Croatia, Czechia, France, Germany, Ireland, Italy, Poland, Portugal, Romania, Spain and the UK (Desvars-Larrive, 2020, p. 3).

In view of the proliferation of COVID-19 policy trackers, a team of researchers in the Department of Social Policy and Intervention at the University of Oxford created a global online directory of relevant policy trackers (Daly et al., 2020). Their supertracker was designed, among others, to facilitate the triangulation of multi-dimensional data from different sources by resolving issues of comparability, coverage and policy impact.

Since the Vienna team's coverage of EU member states is more limited, and the supertracker was not yet operational, Table 3.2 combines scores from the Oxford team's stringency index for three datapoints with information about the absolute numbers of confirmed daily COVID-19 deaths at those dates. Friday 15 May is selected rather than Sunday 17 May (as in Table 2.2) to avoid data reporting issues for deaths occurring during the weekend (Burn-Murdoch, 2020).

At 1 April, Croatia, Italy, Cyprus, France and Slovenia were implementing the most stringent policy measures (Table 3.2). Only Italy and France reported correspondingly high numbers of deaths on that date. The countries operating the least stringent measures were Sweden, Finland and Latvia, matching their relatively low numbers of deaths. Of the other countries reporting relatively large numbers of deaths (Belgium, the Netherlands, Spain and the UK), Spain was closer to the more stringent grouping.

On 1 May 2020, the lockdown rollback checklist showed that only Croatia, Slovakia and Slovenia met almost all the WHO criteria, followed by Greece and Romania (Hale et al., 2020). Another eight member states passed the 50% threshold. The UK, Sweden and Germany fell below 50%.

By 15 May, the stringency index readings had fallen markedly in all countries, except Ireland, Poland and Sweden. The reading for Ireland had risen

Table 3.2 Stringency index and confirmed daily COVID-19 deaths, 1 April, 15 May and 1 July 2020

	1 April		15 May		1 July	
	Stringency	*Deaths*	*Stringency*	*Deaths*	*Stringency*	*Deaths*
Austria	85.19	20	59.26	2	43.52	2
Belgium	81.48	249	75.00	37	42.59	3
Bulgaria	71.30	0	62.96	3	38.89	3
Croatia	96.30	0	70.37	0	36.11	0
Cyprus	92.59	1	92.59	0	60.19	0
Czechia	82.41	7	54.63	3	35.19	1
Denmark	72.22	13	65.74	4	62.96	1
Estonia	77.78	1	55.56	1	22.22	0
Finland	60.19	4	50.93	3	29.63	0
France	90.74	499	76.85	351	52.78	18
Germany	73.15	149	64.35	101	55.09	10
Greece	84.26	6	68.52	1	42.59	1
Hungary	76.85	4	62.96	6	52.78	2
Ireland	85.19	17	90.74	9	38.89	2
Italy	93.52	839	62.96	262	55.56	13
Latvia	65.74	0	62.96	0	46.30	0
Lithuania	81.48	0	75.00	0	35.19	1
Luxembourg	79.63	1	56.48	0	24.07	0
Malta	nd	0	nd	0	nd	0
Netherlands	79.63	175	68.52	28	39.81	2
Poland	81.48	2	83.33	22	50.93	13
Portugal	82.41	20	75.75	9	67.13	5
Romania	87.04	25	72.22	30	50.93	16
Slovakia	75.00	0	73.15	0	40.07	0
Slovenia	89.81	2	53.24	0	33.33	0
Spain	85.19	849	83.33	138	33.80	5
Sweden	40.74	34	46.30	69	40.74	25
UK	75.93	382	69.44	428	71.30	115

Sources: Our World in Data (2020c): daily confirmed deaths; Oxford Blavatnik School of Government (n.d.b): stringency index.

despite a fall in the number of deaths. Spain, France and Belgium also continued to operate stringent measures, despite falling death tolls. By 1 July, the date when most countries had reduced the stringency of their lockdown policy measures, the UK, followed by Portugal, Denmark, Cyprus, Italy, Germany and France, was operating the most stringent measures. The UK's stringency indicator had fluctuated relatively little during the period, while the number of deaths reported remained persistently high. Spain had joined the group with the least stringent measures. Sweden's low stringency level remained almost unchanged throughout the pandemic, despite fluctuations in the number of deaths. In some cases, the countries that had reported death rates close to zero throughout the period had maintained relatively strict lockdown measures, whereas others had been much less stringent, confirming the need to take account of other factors in assessing the relationship between stringency and lethality.

Lifting travel bans

Having been unable to coordinate the introduction of policy measures across the EU, the European Commission sought to encourage a more coordinated response for lifting lockdown, at least as far as the opening of borders was concerned. The process was monitored by Politico EU (2020a) and the Euractiv Network (Brzozowski, 2020), an independent pan-European media network specialising in EU policies. Politico EU and Euractiv found that 15 June was the most popular date for resuming intra-European flights between EU member states.

Ireland, Luxembourg, the Netherlands, Sweden and the UK had never completely suspended travel within the EU when the pandemic was at its peak. Ireland maintained quarantining for most travellers except from Northern Ireland, and the UK introduced it for EU member states as they reported new COVID-19 outbreaks. Most governments announced that they would be prepared to reinstitute targeted lockdown to avoid transmission of the disease.

Observing that 'nearly every member state is playing by its own timetable and rules', Euractiv identified four clusters of countries as they removed travel bans: 'early birds', 'on-timers', 'latecomers' and 'undesirables' (Brzozowski, 2020). Estonia, Latvia and Lithuania were the early birds creating a 'Baltic travel bubble'. They were joined by Poland, Hungary, Croatia, Slovenia and Bulgaria. Although most of the on-timers had also begun lifting travel bans earlier, Austria, France and Germany did not remove restrictions until 15 June. Belgium lifted all restrictions on entry but still faced restrictions on travel to other countries due to its high COVID-19 death rates. Romania maintained bans on travellers from Italy, Spain and Sweden, as did Finland for Sweden. The Netherlands identified 16 member states that it was deemed safe to visit. Travellers to the country had to self-isolate on arrival while they were being tested.

Among the latecomers, Spain postponed opening its borders with other member states until 21 June, and until 1 July for Portugal, but Germans were allowed to travel to the Balearic Islands for a trial period from 15 June. Greece blacklisted visitors from Belgium, France, Italy and the Netherlands until 1 July, and quarantined those arriving from regions with high COVID-19 death rates. Cyprus maintained a few restrictions after reopening to most countries on 20 June. Denmark opted to isolate itself voluntarily until 1 September, with exceptions for visitors from Germany, Finland and Sweden in specified circumstances. Sweden was treated as undesirable due to its 'unconventional pandemic strategy'. The UK was not included in the Euractiv list but might well have belonged to this cluster.

Comparing the economic and social outcomes of lockdown

This overview of the measures taken by governments to suppress or mitigate the spread of the virus, the timing and stringency of their responses, and their preparedness for exiting lockdown has been hampered by the same problems as those encountered elsewhere in this study: the lack of precise, consistent and reliable information and the failure of EU institutions to coordinate interventions. Some patterning across clusters of countries begins to emerge from the analysis of the speed, sequencing and intensity with which different combinations of measures were put in place and the severity of their application. These patterns do not enable meaningful predictions to be made of the overall effectiveness of specific measures. Nor do they explain why individual measures may appear to have been more or less effective in controlling the spread of the virus within or between regions.

The evidence presented in the chapter suggests that some of the socio-demographic characteristics and health indicators that were found in Chapter 2 to influence the spread of the pandemic may also contribute to an understanding of the findings in this chapter. Smaller less densely populated countries with relatively well-resourced health services, less dependence on international connectivity, and the capacity to exercise tighter control over the behaviour of their populations, would appear to be in a better position to stem the spread of the virus.

Online tools tracking developments across most, if not all, member states have proved to be valuable not only for informing policy but also for identifying clustering of countries and potential outliers in a constantly evolving landscape. Their findings help to raise awareness of the complex task facing the European Commission as it attempted to fulfil its treaty obligations by ensuring a high level of human health protection, coordinating action between member states and cooperating with them to prevent diseases and combat cross-border threats to health, while leaving member states responsible for the organisation and delivery of public health policies.

Note

1 The European Commission president, Ursula von der Leyen, could be watched on YouTube demonstrating hand washing while humming the EU's anthem, 'Ode to joy'. https://www.youtube.com/watch?v=sLa_QiWulPE

4   The impact of COVID-19 in policy contexts

This chapter examines the ways in which EU member states dealt with the COVID-19 pandemic by setting information about the spread of the virus and the mitigation strategies adopted by governments at international, national and local levels in the context of their policy environments and the policymaking process. The chapter looks behind the headlines and statistics to explore the relationship between state power and public attitudes towards government interventions, drawing on data about public trust in politicians and scientists, to identify similarities and differences in policy responses and their impact on social and economic life. Fluctuations in public opinion and perceptions of government interventions are found to affect policy outcomes. The chapter shows how knowledge about the diversity of policy environments, administrative cultures and legislative frameworks in different countries can contribute to a better understanding of the performance of national governments and EU institutions in dealing with COVID-19 and preparing for future outbreaks of the pandemic. The conclusion reviews the impact of the pandemic on administrative structures and legal processes in different policy contexts.

Policy environments and the policymaking process

From the onset of the pandemic, national governments exercised their responsibility for making and implementing public health policy in accordance with their own healthcare systems and political competences. Differences in funding arrangements, levels and modes of service provision, as well as protective capacity suggested that individual member states were not equally well equipped, either financially or logistically, to confront a global crisis (Chapter 1). Socio-demographic factors contributed to the challenges governments faced in containing or suppressing the spread of COVID-19 (Chapter 2). The decision-making process was further complicated by the uncertainties surrounding the disease and the lack of a reliable and consensual scientific evidence base with which to inform policy. Governments were also hampered by the national and international policy environments in which they operate. Many EU member states were still recovering from the 2008 global economic crisis, and from the ensuing wave of political turbulence that had swept across Europe, exacerbated by the refugee crisis in 2015 and the UK's decision to leave the EU in 2016 (Hantrais, 2019). Following a series of extreme weather events, and in the wake of the Extinction Rebellion protests, by late 2019 global climate change was high on EU and national political agendas. Many member states had recently held legislative elections or were about to do so. The UK had just negotiated its formal exit from the EU on 31 January 2020 when COVID-19 struck. The already-weakened resilience of governments and the public at large was to be sorely tested by the pandemic.

The EU policy context

The UK entered the transition phase of negotiations with a newly installed European Commission, Parliament, Council presidency and several recently elected heads of state or government. Arguably, the COVID-19 pandemic was the greatest challenge that the EU had to face in its 63 years of existence. EU institutions had to decide how they would exercise their mandate for ensuring a high level of human health protection, coordinating action between member states and promoting research into the causes and transmission of 'major health scourges' (Article 168, 2007 Lisbon Treaty). Like many governments in member states (COVID–DEM Infohub, 2020), the Commission was criticised for its initial delay in reacting to the pandemic. Subsequently, member states accused the Commission of acting too fast and for exceeding its legal powers.

In the early stages of the pandemic, like the World Health Organisation (WHO), the Commission hesitated to acknowledge publicly the seriousness of the outbreak. The failure of EU heads of state or government, in their capacity as members of the European Council, to reach agreement over the 2021–27 EU budget at their meeting in February 2020 exposed latent divisions, reflecting their different approaches to governance and foreshadowing their varying policy responses to the pandemic. At its videoconference on 10 March, the European Council (2020a) recognised the situation as an integrated policy crisis emergency, severely challenging EU solidarity and justifying a centrally coordinated response. But Council members were unable to agree, then or subsequently, on a concerted collegiate strategy. Despite the apparent unity expressed in the summit's conclusions, national leaders disagreed over how to contain the pandemic without causing irreparable damage to their economies, a fundamental dilemma that was to persist over the coming weeks and months.

A few days later, on 13 March when WHO (2020d) identified the EU as the epicentre of the pandemic, governments in EU member states were already responding by unilaterally applying protective and preventative measures with greater or lesser degrees of stringency, and in line with national circumstances and priorities (Chapter 3). One of the core conditions for EU membership, free movement of people, over which the EU's Brexit negotiators remained adamant, was the first of the EU's red lines to be widely flouted as member states closed their internal borders. Rather than being proactive, the European Commission (2020, 16 March) reacted by attempting to persuade member states (including the UK) to focus on EU's external borders to protect the Single Market. Paradoxically, the UK kept its borders open, but so did Ireland, France, Luxembourg and Malta.

While remaining within the Commission's statutory mandate, its president, Ursula von der Leyen, announced a European instrument for temporary Support to mitigate Unemployment Risks in an Emergency (SURE) (European Commission, 2020, 2 April). The EU's structural funds were to be deployed to support short-time work schemes in member states. To leverage the financial power of SURE, loans were provided on favourable terms, underpinned by guarantees voluntarily committed to by member states based on their contribution to the EU budget. The Commission promoted the scheme as an essential source of social support for furloughed workers and their families at risk of poverty, in effect providing a social protection floor. SURE required the relaxation of rules on state aid and the suspension of strict regulations on public deficits in the eurozone countries, reflecting the Commission's awareness of the need to adopt a conciliatory approach if member states were to accept the scheme. The Commission was reminded of the importance of exercising caution in the performance of its mandate when, on 7 April, news was leaked that a proposed roadmap for exiting lockdown would be adopted the following day. The evening headlines announced: 'Governments force Commission into U-turn over fears it was moving too quickly' (Bayer, 2020).

Rather than proceeding with the roadmap at that time, the European Commission (2020, 8 April) adopted a communication setting out formal guidelines to optimise the supply and availability of medicines across the EU, including the UK. Having already announced the creation of a strategic 'rescEU stockpile' of medical equipment such as ventilators and protective masks (European Commission, 2020, 19 March), the Communication advocated direct emergency support for national healthcare sectors. Member states were advised to support the manufacturing capacity of industry using fiscal incentives and state aid. Advice was proffered on personal protective equipment (PPE), cross-border movement of goods and workers, monitoring of national stocks and flexibility in public procurement.

As in 2008 following the financial crisis, this time using its public health treaty mandate, the European Commission (2020, 27 May) prepared a detailed recovery plan. Next Generation EU focussed on mitigating the effects of COVID-19 and supporting 'a fair and inclusive recovery'. The plan built on the Commission's Green Deal, which had been retained as a priority and had gained momentum during lockdown, while addressing lessons that could be drawn from the crisis. Despite the Commission's cautious approach, initial responses to the proposal from national governments again exposed the underlying lack of unity and solidarity among EU member states, raising constitutional concerns about the EU's legal integrity (Alemanno, 2020).

National administrative cultures

When the European Economic Community was founded in 1957, together the six original member states totalled 167 million inhabitants. On 1 January 2020, with 28 member states, the EU's population reached 445 million. In the early years of the EEC, consensus was not easily achieved, given the diversity of interests, power structures and economic resources of the founding member states. The 22 new countries that progressively joined the EU in the five subsequent waves of membership (Table 4.1) brought with them an ever greater variety of social, economic and political structures and traditions,

Table 4.1 EU (by wave), Schengen and eurozone membership, administrative performance, 2017, quality of democracy, 2019

Country	EU wave	Schengen	Eurozone	Administration score	Democracy score	Health policy score
Austria	4	x	x	12	7.4	7
Belgium	1	x	x	14	7.3	7
Bulgaria	6	–	–	28	5.6	4
Croatia	6	–	–	28	5.7	4
Cyprus	5	–	x	26	6.2	6
Czechia	5	x	–	22	5.7	7
Denmark	2	x	–	6	8.9	8
Estonia	5	x	x	11	8.7	8
Finland	4	x	x	6	9.1	7
France	1	x	x	15	7.2	7
Germany	1	x	x	15	8.7	8
Greece	3	x	x	29	6.8	4
Hungary	5	x	–	26	3.4	3
Ireland	2	–	x	13	8.2	5
Italy	1	x	x	25	7.2	7
Latvia	5	x	x	17	7.9	4
Lithuania	5	x	x	17	8.1	7
Luxembourg	1	x	x	13	7.6	8
Malta	5	x	x	16	5.7	7
Netherlands	1	x	x	9	7.3	6
Poland	5	x	–	19	5.1	5
Portugal	3	x	x	19	7.5	6
Romania	6	–	–	29	4.9	4
Slovakia	5	x	x	26	6.5	4
Slovenia	5	x	x	23	7.3	5
Spain	3	x	x	19	7.3	8
Sweden	4	x	–	7	9.3	6
UK	2	–	–	10	7.3	6

Sources: Bertelmann Stiftung (2019a, 2019b): democracy and health policy scores (10 = highest); Thijs et al. (2018, graph 40): administration scores (6 = highest).

making the prospects of achieving the goal of closer political union ever more distant.

Within the EU, in addition to extending the array of statutory treaty commitments, most EU member states signed up to the Schengen agreement, which regulated the number of asylum seekers entering EU member states and protected the EU's external borders (Table 4.1). Other member states met the conditions for joining the eurozone, thereby ceding control over national and economic monetary policy to the European Central Bank. Denmark negotiated an opt-out from the eurozone, and Sweden avoided fulfilling the adoption requirements. The UK had declined to join both Schengen and the eurozone, in line with its reputation for being 'half in half out' of the EU (Adonis, 2018). Membership of Schengen and the eurozone did not prevent like-minded member states from forming pressure groups around specific issues and during times of crisis, as exemplified by the 2008 financial and 2015 refugee crises (Hantrais, 2019), and as would be further illustrated during the COVID-19 crisis in their reactions to Commission proposals for economic recovery (Chapter 5).

By taking the chair of the rotating presidency of the Council for six months, according to a prescribed order, in theory member states have an opportunity to influence the legislative agenda, and to play a lead role in dealing with the latest crisis. Estonia occupied this position when it replaced the UK in July 2017 following the Brexit referendum. Croatia, the most recent member of the EU (neither in Schengen nor the eurozone), held the presidency when Europe became the epicentre of the COVID-19 pandemic; Croatia was succeeded by Germany in July 2020. The decision in 2009 (Article 15, Lisbon Treaty) to appoint an elected president of the European Council for a longer term of office (2.5×2 years) substantially reduced the powers of the rotating presidency. In 2020, Donald Tusk from Poland was replaced in that position by Charles Michel, who had previously served as prime minister of Belgium. Michel was actively involved in chairing EU summit meetings during the pandemic crisis, while Croatia maintained a low profile and attracted little media attention.

Arguably, how governments responded to the pandemic by introducing and lifting lockdowns (Chapter 3), the degree to which the public complied with restrictions and the effectiveness of the policy measures implemented depended on a combination of factors: state traditions, the characteristics of their public administrations and the nature of the relationship between the state and its electorate (Box 4.1).

Box 4.1 Public administration and democracy indicators

As part of a project commissioned by the Directorate-General for Employment, Social Affairs and Inclusion on 'Support for developing better country knowledge on public administration and institutional capacity building', Thijs et al. (2018) conducted a study of 'Key characteristics of public administration in member states'. The research team undertook a substantive overview of public administration systems, cultures and functions in the years before the pandemic. Their indicator-based assessment of both capacity and performance of public administration covered five dimensions: transparency and accountability; civil service systems and human resource management; service delivery and digitalisation; organisation and management of government; and policymaking, coordination and implementation. The authors stressed the importance of contextual knowledge for a valid interpretation of their indicators by referring to country-specific features of public administration at the time when the study was conducted. They used aggregated scores, based on the quintile assessment for different dimensions of public administration, to produce an indicator of overall performance. The best possible aggregated score is 6, while a maximum score of 30 means that a country was always ranked in the lowest quintile.

The study by Thijs et al. (2018, p. 13, annex 2) included information about multi-level governance. They showed that most EU member states have two or three administrative tiers. Austria, Belgium, France, Germany, Italy, Poland and Spain have four, and Portugal has five. Although federal states in the EU have an overarching unitary state structure, Germany is depicted as a 'fully-fledged federation' and Austria as a 'centralised federal State'. Belgium, Spain and the UK were 'characterised by asymmetries between regional and state governments in terms of competences'. Provision of services, including public utilities and health policy, is largely shared between the different levels of government.

The Bertelmann Stiftung (2019b), an independent foundation supporting projects contributing to social reform, combined qualitative assessments and quantitative data to compile a series of indicators covering policy performance, democracy and governance in OECD and EU countries. Their sustainable governance indicators (SGIs) were designed to assist stakeholders in navigating the complexity of effective governance in answer to a question that underpins the analysis throughout this book: What works in which context and why? The components in their composite indicator for quality of democracy – electoral processes, access to information, civil rights and political liberties, and rule of law – were equally weighted (25%). The highest possible score for this indicator is 10.

The Bertelmann Stiftung's (2019a) health performance indicators covered health policy (weighted 50%), spending on preventive health programmes, perceived health status, life expectancy and infant mortality (each weighted 12.5%). They were looking for evidence of high-quality, inclusive and efficient healthcare provision at the lowest possible costs. Of the three criteria, efficiency was given less weight if the first two criteria were fulfilled. The highest possible score for this indicator is 10.

The COVID–DEM Infohub (n.d.) was established in 2020 under the auspices of Democracy Reporting International, a non-partisan, independent, not-for-profit organisation registered in Berlin. The hub's mission was to help democracy analysts track, compile and share information on how state responses to COVID-19 are impacting on democratic governance. The 142 country reports from a 50-day Symposium in April/May 2020 provide granular analyses by lawyers of the varied government responses to the pandemic in EU member states (COVID–DEM Infohub, 2020). These reports can be used to assess how, in practice, democratic governments and their administrations performed during the crisis.

In their assessment of administrative performance Thijs et al. (2018) attributed the highest scores to Denmark, Finland and Sweden (Table 4.1). A second cluster of countries performed relatively well: the Netherlands, the UK, Estonia, Austria, Ireland, Luxembourg, France and Germany. At the other end of the scale, Romania, Greece, Croatia, Bulgaria, Slovakia, Hungary, Cyprus and Italy, in that order, were identified as the member states in greatest need of administrative improvement.

Despite the different components in the composite indicators for quality of democracy, the Bertelmann Stiftung's (2019b) indicators for policy performance in EU member states identified a similar, but not identical, clustering of countries to that produced by Thijs et al. (2018) for administrative performance (Table 4.1). Sweden, Finland and Denmark maintained their positions at the top of the rank order, where they were joined by Germany and Ireland. Bulgaria and Romania remained at the bottom, where they were joined by Poland and Hungary. The Netherlands, the UK, France and Austria displayed lower rankings for democratic indicators than for administrative capacity.

The Bertelmann Stiftung (2019a) found that Denmark, Germany, Estonia and Luxembourg largely met their criteria for health policy, scoring 8 out of 10 for this indicator. The criteria were only partly achieved in Ireland, Poland and Slovenia, with a score of 5. The performance of Bulgaria, Croatia and Greece, Latvia, Romania and Slovakia was deemed to be inadequate, while healthcare policy in Hungary, with 3, was described as one of the most 'conflict-ridden' policy fields.

These different sets of indicators did not enable accurate predictions of how governments would perform during the COVID-19 crisis. In conjunction with information about other aspects of political and administrative cultures, they contribute to a better understanding of how the decision-making process was subsequently adapted to meet the unprecedented challenges facing governments in 2020.

Administrative performance during the pandemic

Any comparison of administrative performance across the EU during the pandemic needs to take account of the ways in which powers were distributed and used not only between parliament, government and the executive, but also between different levels of national, regional and local governance (Table 4.2). The international standing of national leaders in their capacity as members of the European Council also has a bearing on the decision-making process and its effectiveness.

In his overview of the impact of the pandemic on democratic practices in the countries participating in the COVID–DEM Infohub, Daly (2020) observed that, from a lawyer's perspective, 'An unprecedented number of states have derogated *en masse* from international human rights treaties and are simultaneously under a state of emergency (or emergency measures without a formal emergency declaration)'. Noting that COVID-19 responses are 'starkly uneven across democracies worldwide', Daly identified four broad categories of governments: effective or constrained rationalists, autocratic opportunists and fantasists. He named Hungary as a prime example of an autocratic opportunist. Poland was cited as a case where 'the pandemic has simply laid bare the true nature of the political system'. Sweden and the UK were referred to as countries where 'their already sullied democratic reputations' have been further tarnished.

In her introduction to the Symposium, Grogan (2020b) cites several EU member states to illustrate the different approaches adopted in managing the crisis, and their success, or failure, in limiting the potential for abuse and containing the pandemic. The country reports published on the COVID–DEM Infohub (2020) show how the pandemic continuously tested and challenged the constitutional limits of what Daly (2020) describes as 'overreaching governmental action', even in countries that did not declare a formal state of emergency or institute special emergency powers. The great diversity exhibited by EU member states in other aspects of governance is abundantly demonstrated by the different ways in which they used legal instruments to manage their responses to the pandemic (Box 4.2).

Box 4.2 Diversity of legal instruments

Some governments introduced a state of emergency, either as provided for in their constitutions or by creating new statutes (Table 3.1).

Some countries did not declare a state of emergency, because their constitutions did not make the necessary provision, because they did not want to embark on that route for historical reasons, or because their ordinary legislation already contained sufficient powers.

Eleven EU member states declared 'a state of emergency' between 16 and 31 March. The constitutions in a few countries already contained provision for health emergencies. Portugal had a Law of Civic Protection, a Framework Health Law and a Law on Public Vigilance of Health Risks. Other member states created new statutes: Czechia instituted a Crisis Management Act, Estonia a highly prescriptive Emergency Act, Finland an Emergency Powers Act, France an Emergency Response to the COVID-19 Epidemic Act, Slovakia a COVID-19 Emergency Act and Poland a COVID-19 Statute, which was deemed by lawyers to be unconstitutional (Jaraczewski, 2020). Austria, which instituted an Epidemic Diseases Act and a COVID-19 Measures Act, was described as having a statutory, but not a constitutional, state of emergency (Lachmayer, 2020). Hungary's Enabling Act went well beyond a state of emergency, in effect giving the government a parliamentary mandate to act by decree without parliamentary scrutiny or a sunset law (Kovács, 2020). Romania later replaced its state of emergency by a 'state of alert' as part of its exit plan (Selejan-Gutan, 2020), while Spain declared a 'state of alarm' (Ángel Presno Linera, 2020).

Without declaring a state of emergency, Malta instituted an Emergency Powers Act, Ireland a Health Act as well as an Emergency Act, Denmark an Epidemics Act and the UK a Coronavirus Act 2020, although its Public Health (Control of Diseases) Act already allowed for restrictions on movement (Grogan, 2020a). The Irish courts were prepared to stretch the meaning of the Constitution to accommodate exceptional powers without the need to declare an actual state of emergency (Greene, 2020). Croatia, Denmark, the Netherlands and Sweden relied on existing statutory frameworks. Germany integrated extraordinary powers, or 'interventions' in the regular legal framework of political decision-making (Jürgensen & Orlowski, 2020). Lithuania, which, like Germany, debated whether to declare a state of emergency, added a Quarantine Resolution to an already crowded statute book containing a Law on State of Emergency, a Law on Civil Protection and a Law on the Prevention and Control of Contagious Diseases (Dagilytė et al., 2020). Exceptional powers were almost always time limited, but with provision for extensions. Their duration varied from 10 days in Luxembourg, 15 days in Italy and Spain, 1 month in France, 30 days in Czechia, Denmark and Romania, to 90 days in Slovakia and 6 months in the UK.

Table 4.2 Political systems in EU member states

Country	Government	Unitary/federal	Monarchy/republic	Head of state/ EU Council	Head of government/EU Council
Austria	Parliamentary	Federal	Republic	Federal President	**Federal Chancellor**
Belgium	Parliamentary	Federal	Monarchy	King	**Prime Minister**
Bulgaria	Parliamentary	Unitary	Republic	President	**Minister–Chairman**
Croatia	Parliamentary	Unitary	Republic	President	**Prime Minister**
Cyprus	Semi-presidential	Unitary	Republic	**President**	**President**
Czechia	Parliamentary	Unitary	Republic	President	**Prime Minister**
Denmark	Parliamentary	Federate	Monarchy	Queen	**Minister of State**
Estonia	Parliamentary	Unitary	Republic	President	**Prime Minister**
Finland	Parliamentary	Federate	Republic	President	**Prime Minister**
France	Semi-presidential	Federate	Republic	**President**	Prime Minister
Germany	Parliamentary	Federal	Republic	Federal President	**Federal Chancellor**
Greece	Parliamentary	Unitary	Republic	President	**Prime Minister**
Hungary	Parliamentary	Unitary	Republic	President	**Prime Minister**
Ireland	Parliamentary	Unitary	Republic	President	**Taoiseach**
Italy	Parliamentary	Devolved	Republic	President	**Prime Minister**
Latvia	Parliamentary	Unitary	Republic	President	**Prime Minister**
Lithuania	Semi-presidential	Unitary	Republic	**President**	Minister-President
Luxembourg	Parliamentary	Unitary	Monarchy	Grand Duke	**Prime Minister**
Malta	Parliamentary	Unitary	Republic	President	**Prime Minister**
Netherlands	Parliamentary	Federate	Monarchy	King	**Prime Minister**
Poland	Semi-presidential	Unitary	Republic	President	**Prime Minister**
Portugal	Semi-presidential	Unitary	Republic	President	**Prime Minister**
Romania	Semi-presidential	Unitary	Republic	**President**	Prime Minister
Slovakia	Parliamentary	Unitary	Republic	President	**Prime Minister**
Slovenia	Parliamentary	Unitary	Republic	President	**Prime Minister**
Spain	Parliamentary	Devolved	Monarchy	King	**Prime Minister**
Sweden	Parliamentary	Unitary	Monarchy	King	**Prime Minister**
UK	Parliamentary	Unitary/devolved	Monarchy	Queen	**Prime Minister**

Sources: European Council/Council of the European Union (2020); Wikipedia (n.d.a).

In addition to their varied legal bases, the stability or fragility of the government at the time of the crisis complicated the decision-making process and the effectiveness of the measures enacted. Several member states held legislative or presidential elections in 2019, during the pandemic or as lockdown was being lifted, often resulting in changes of government or leadership and creating conflicts both within governments and between legislative and executive powers (Box 4.3).

Box 4.3 Changing distribution of legislative and executive powers

In 2019, elections had been held in Austria, Greece, Poland, Portugal, Romania, Spain and the UK (Institute for Government, 2020). Greece saw a shift to a right-wing opposition party. The UK had replaced its prime minister and held a general election in December, which produced a working majority for the Conservatives. The general election in Spain brought to power a left-wing PSOE−Podemos coalition. Elections in Italy produced a coalition between the centre-left Democratic Party and the populist Five Star Movement. In Slovenia, the onset of the pandemic coincided with a shift in power, as the prime minister resigned, and a new coalition was hastily built to avoid the need for a snap election; the transition gave a caretaker government authority to declare a state of emergency (Zagorc & Bardutzky, 2020). When the EU became the epicentre of the pandemic, Belgium had been ruled by a caretaker government for 15 months. When Croatia assumed the rotating presidency of the EU, it had just elected a new president. On 22 March 2020, the government had to deal with an additional emergency when an earthquake hit Zagreb. In the presidential elections spread across 2019 and 2020, the centre-left candidate beat the incumbent centre-right candidate. In the general elections that took place in July after Croatia passed on the EU presidency to Germany, the incumbent centre-right party increased its majority in recognition of its management of the crises.

Slovakian politics were emerging from a heated campaign in the run-up to general elections on 29 February 2020 (Henčeková & Drugda, 2020). The shift that took place from a centre-left to a centre-right government meant that the newly elected government, without the benefit of experience, had to respond to calls for strong and decisive measures to contain the pandemic. The elections in Ireland in February resulted in a coalition government, with the Fine Gael leader temporarily remaining as Taioseach (Greene, 2020), to be replaced in June by a Fianna Fáil leader. For Romania, 2020 was again an electoral year affecting the ability of the government to manage the crisis: political conflicts between the parliament, government and executive increased (Selejan-Gutan, 2020). Poland was in dispute with the European Commission regarding the independence of the Polish Supreme Court (Jaraczewski, 2020). The actions taken by the Polish government to curb the powers of the courts rendered the Polish Constitutional Tribunal 'nonfunctional' as a guardian of human rights, to the extent that it became 'a hollow shell of its former self, completely taken over by the ruling party'. In July 2020, Poland's incumbent president narrowly beat the challenger, meaning that the governing PiS party would be able to pursue the controversial policies that had brought him into conflict with the EU.

Despite marked differences in COVID-19 transmission rates not only between countries but also within them (Chapter 2), in the early stages of the epidemic, most countries imposed national lockdowns (Chapter 3). In the absence of adequate testing regimes, centralised governments were tasked with managing the distribution of equipment and other resources that were often in short supply. As within the EU, the responsibility for health is a shared competence within countries; administrative responsibility for delivering services is usually delegated to regional and local levels (Boxes 4.1 and 4.4). Depending on the degree of coordination, the sharing of powers either contributed to administrative efficiency or created mixed messaging and regulatory confusion, not least for mobile workers both within and between countries and regions.

Box 4.4 Central and regional distribution of powers

In Germany, with its strong federal structure, the Disaster Protection Act was implemented by the *Länder* (Jürgensen & Orlowski, 2020). They had the power to decide when and how to ease lockdown, which created 'frustration in Berlin as some states lift curbs ahead of conference aimed at co-ordinating strategy' (Chazan, 2020). The COVID-19 Measures Act in Austria empowered the Minister of Health as well as regional and local health authorities to ban the access to certain (defined) places (Lachmayer, 2020). The 'asymmetries between regional and state governments in terms of competences' (Thijs et al., 2018) proved to be an advantage in Belgium by providing a safety net for the rule of law and avoiding the risk of abuses that could have arisen under powerful centralised government control (Ganty, 2020). In Spain, tensions emerged between central and regional authorities over the management of the pandemic (Ángel Presno Linera, 2020). Despite its decentralised structure, measures were not negotiated with the autonomous regions, but central government was forced to allow their participation in decisions about easing lockdown. In the UK, where health is devolved to the nations, the power to decide on the timing and scope of measures meant that England, Northern Ireland, Scotland and Wales announced the imposition and easing of lockdown on different dates, causing friction with central government and mixed messaging.

The Netherlands used the powers of their Public Health Act to instruct mayors to issue emergency regulations, but the government rapidly decided that it would need to intervene to coordinate and harmonise the regulations to prevent people moving from one part of the country to another with 'lighter' rules (Buyse, & de Lange, 2020). In Italy, where COVID-19 cases clustered in Lombardy and Veneto, legislative and administrative measures were passed and enforced at different levels (national, regional and local), resulting in the need for decree-laws to correct 'ambiguity regarding the geographical scope of the measures', and to avoid the 'legal chaos' created by the government's initially hasty uncoordinated response (Beqiraj, 2020). In Portugal, the complexity of the enabling framework led to centralisation of power to the executive (Violante & Lanceiro, 2020). In Sweden, at national level, the parliament and government determined the goals to be achieved using basic rules and binding statutes on standards (Cameron & Jonsson-Cornell, 2020). Responsibility for hospital and primary healthcare was devolved to the regions, but the municipalities retained responsibility for the care of older people and those with physical and mental disabilities.

Irrespective of whether or not a state of emergency had been declared, the proportionality, and hence legality, of the measures imposed using different legislative instruments was contested in the courts, unless they had been suspended, and by the wider public (Box 4.5). Particular concerns were raised in most member states about measures that restricted freedom of movement (travel bans, quarantine), assembly (religious practice and ceremonies) and other forms of association (gatherings and events), and the right to family/ private life (visits to relations in care homes, attendance of fathers at childbirths) (Chapter 3).

Box 4.5 Proportionality of government measures

Fears were widespread about the proportionality of measures that required access to virtual healthcare and education (e-health, distance learning, teleworking); curtailed democratic processes (holding elections, legal scrutiny of legislation); and enabled surveillance of private life by making provision for the transfer of personal data (electronic tracking and tracing of infected persons, 'smart' quarantining).

By closing down ordinary courts, the Hungarian government used its extraordinary powers to prevent review of the measures introduced, potentially shifting the balance of power permanently to executive decision-making (Kovács, 2020). In Czechia, although the Constitutional Court annulled some restrictive measures introduced by the Ministry of Health, it lacked the competence to review the declaration of the state of emergency (Vikarská, 2020). In Romania, neither Parliament nor the Constitutional Court was competent to review the presidential decree instituting the state of emergency (Selejan-Gutan, 2020). In Latvia, under the constitution, sittings of parliament had to take place in Riga; video conferences were conducted remotely, with members of parliament in different parts of the building (Dimitrovs, 2020).

Doubts were expressed in France about the amount of trust that could be placed in the administrative courts in general, and the Council of State, 'to be thorough defenders of public liberties' (Platon, 2020). The Finnish and Bulgarian governments were criticised for their lack of legal and constitutional expertise (Scheinin, 2020; Vassileva, 2020); and the commission of legal experts operating within Croatia's Ministry of Health was reproached for its 'smokescreen of expertise' (Bačić Selanec, 2020). At times, as exemplified by Cyprus and Estonia, it was difficult to discern whether policies were implemented to further party political agendas or the public good (Laulhé Shaelou & Manoli, 2020; Maruste, 2020). The Greek government proved to be capable of exploiting the 'plasticity of the proportionality principle' to ease doubts about the conformity of the emergency measures with the Greek Constitution (Karavokyris, 2020).

Whereas Portugal gave assurances that no restrictions on freedom of expression and press freedom would be allowed during the crisis (Violante & Lanceiro, 2020), in Hungary and Romania, emergency powers were used to restrict freedom of expression. The Enabling Act in Hungary introduced 'rules to curb the remaining free press further by criminalising the obstruction of epidemiological control and the publication of false or distorted facts that interfere with the "successful protection" of the public' (Kovács, 2020). In Romania, the Prosecutor's Office opened investigations against doctors in a state hospital designated to treat COVID-19 patients because they had publicly complained about lack of equipment (Selejan-Gutan, 2020).

Although, under international law, governments can derogate to human rights in circumstances of public emergency, they must ensure that the measures they adopt do not disproportionally harm vulnerable people (Lebret, 2020). Concerns were widely voiced, for example in Finland, Latvia, Lithuania, Luxembourg, Poland, Portugal, Spain and the UK, not only about the pandemic's impact on public health but also about the effects of lockdown measures on the lives of the most vulnerable groups. Arguably, women and children in dysfunctional and abusive households, disabled and older people with underlying health conditions, and low-income groups were being exposed to politically unacceptable risks of poverty, economic and social exclusion. Government interventions were criticised for intensifying socio-economic inequalities as digital solutions such as distance learning, online healthcare, teleworking and restrictions on public transport widened social divides and heightened concerns about the invasion of privacy.

Governments and health services were held to account on legal and ethical grounds (Box 4.6). Complaints were registered in many countries about the lack of checks and balances during the state of emergency. Most governments deferred to scientific, legal and constitutional expertise to guide their decisions about the formulation, timing, stringency and proportionality of measures with the aim of enabling legal scrutiny and, thereby, avoiding the accusation of overreaching their legal powers.

Box 4.6 Legal challenges to government powers

Complaints were brought before the administrative courts in Czechia concerning the legality of restrictions on freedom of movement (Vikarská, 2020). The proportionality of penalties was challenged in Romanian courts (Selejan-Gutan, 2020). Lawsuits were brought against governments that had not closed down activities and events in good time, for example the Tyrolean government in Austria after an early outbreak in a ski resort (Lachmayer, 2020). In Italy, public prosecutors opened criminal investigations to determine responsibility for localised outbreaks (Beqiraj, 2020). In France, some 90 complaints had been lodged by individuals, doctors, associations or prisoners against the French government since the beginning of the epidemic for endangering people's lives (Paun, 2020). Investigations were opened in July against the former prime minister and two former ministers of health for abstaining from fighting a disaster. In Lithuania, the activities of a private social care home, a hospital and individuals who left the hospital in spite of suspected COVID-19 were under investigation (Dagilytė et al., 2020). Most of the prohibitions in Poland were hard, legally enforceable orders severely limiting human rights and freedoms

(Jaraczewski, 2020). Flouting them incurred the risk of severe financial penalties. The government introduced disproportionate administrative fines for breach of lockdown orders. By having recourse to administrative rather than criminal measures, it avoided the obligation of a court hearing and the opportunity for defence.

Even though they were relatively unaffected by the pandemic, Cyprus, Estonia, Greece and Hungary took advantage of the COVID-19 crisis to deter illegal migrants from entering their territories, and/or to justify keeping refugees confined in camp lockdowns. Slovakia deployed the military to prevent the spread of the disease into and out of Roma communities (Henčeková & Drugda, 2020). Belgium and Luxembourg, among others, denounced the overcrowded and insanitary conditions in reception facilities during lockdown for endangering the fundamental rights of refugees and denying them access to international protection (Ganty, 2020; Stoppioni, 2020). To offset such concerns, Portugal regularised the situation of migrants by granting them access to fundamental rights such as healthcare, housing and social support (Violante & Lanceiro, 2020).

Public attitudes towards government interventions

To operate efficiently, democratic governments need the support of their citizens. As new outbreaks began to occur, governments became increasingly alert to the need to manage public expectations by using clear and consistent messaging as well as transparency if they were to avoid crisis fatigue. They also recognised the importance of taking account of public opinion if they were to retain popular support and trust, and to ensure that they remained in power.

Eurobarometer surveys conducted in earlier years provide an indication of the amount of trust that the public had in their governments and in EU institutions prior to the COVID-19 crisis. The official show of European unity throughout the negotiation phase of the Brexit Withdrawal Agreement was underpinned by a high level of public support for more EU initiatives to deal with health and social security, as recorded in a Eurobarometer (2017, QC7.2) survey on social issues (Table 4.3). At that time, Cyprus, Belgium, Portugal, Spain and Slovenia strongly supported more decision-making at EU level to deal with health and social security issues. At the other end of the scale, Austria, Finland, Sweden and Denmark were less supportive of EU intervention in these areas. Two years later when Eurobarometer (2019, QA6a.14) published the first results from the autumn survey, trust in the EU was at 43%, 10 points above trust in national governments and parliaments.

Health and social security ranked as the most important issue of national concern in the autumn of 2019 (Table 4.3), at over 40% for respondents in Finland, Hungary, Portugal, Slovakia and Sweden notwithstanding their

Table 4.3 Public opinion in EU member states, 2017, 2019 and 2020

	2017	2019	May 2020	Most trusted information	
	Support for EU	Concern with health	Satisfied with government	Scientists	Government
Austria	46	18	78	37	39
Belgium	76	12	57	51	15
Bulgaria	67	38	46	31	20
Croatia	67	18	68	44	16
Cyprus	83	13	nd	nd	nd
Czechia	57	18	65	38	26
Denmark	42	38	85	37	43
Estonia	53	27	nd	nd	nd
Finland	33	48	79	35	38
France	57	17	42	41	19
Germany	61	17	66	39	25
Greece	61	9	77	58	21
Hungary	68	42	48	32	22
Ireland	63	39	85	31	43
Italy	59	9	55	42	22
Latvia	60	43	nd	nd	nd
Lithuania	64	23	nd	nd	nd
Luxembourg	66	4	nd	nd	nd
Malta	69	2	nd	nd	nd
Netherlands	54	31	81	40	43
Poland	65	28	40	40	10
Portugal	76	44	83	28	24
Romania	68	24	52	34	17
Slovakia	58	45	72	39	24
Slovenia	70	38	54	37	7
Spain	73	13	35	48	18
Sweden	38	41	67	36	28
UK	50	37	nd	nd	nd

Sources: Eurobarometer (2017, p. 48); Eurobarometer (2019, p. 25); European Parliament (2020b, pp. 44, 48).

different welfare systems. The issue ranked second for over 30% of respondents. In Estonia, it shared second place with pensions. Health and social security ranked third in Lithuania, and equal third in Austria along with unemployment and rising prices/inflation/cost of living.

When asked what they thought were the most important issues facing the EU in 2019 (Eurobarometer, 2019, QA5a, p. 19), a third of respondents in all countries except Austria, Ireland and Sweden ranked immigration at the top of the list. When asked for their opinion on reinforcing the EU's external borders (Eurobarometer, 2019, QB6.2, p. 28), more than half of respondents were in favour in every EU member state, indicating that the European Commission could expect its action to be well received when it recommended closing external borders at the onset of the pandemic. Cyprus and Greece (both 91%) and Bulgaria (85%) were most supportive of the proposal in 2019. The UK (55%) and Sweden (57%) were least supportive; the

UK did not close its national borders in March 2020, and Sweden banned only non-essential travel.

The European Parliament (2020b) commissioned a Public Opinion Monitoring Study covering the period between 23 April and 1 May 2020 when COVID-19 restrictions were beginning to be lifted. The fieldwork excluded the smallest EU member states in terms of population size: Lithuania, Estonia, Latvia, Cyprus, Malta and Luxembourg. The UK was not included since it was no longer officially a member of the EU. The findings offer insights into the public mood during the pandemic and indicate the extent to which the public supported the measures taken by their governments. At the time of the survey, Denmark, Ireland, Portugal and the Netherlands recorded satisfaction scores over 80% (Table 4.3). Satisfaction ratings fell below 50% in Hungary, Bulgaria, France, Poland and Spain.

When questioned about what they considered to be trustworthy sources of information on the pandemic, respondents in 12 countries were found to be most likely to believe scientists (Table 4.3). In Denmark, especially, and in Ireland, the Netherlands, Austria and Finland, respondents were most likely to believe national health authorities. In Hungary, Portugal and Romania, they put most trust in the WHO. Only in Denmark, Ireland, the Netherlands, Austria, Finland, Slovakia and Czechia, was the government cited as one of the three most trustworthy sources of information. Respondents in none of the 21 countries surveyed included EU institutions among their three most trustworthy sources of information about the pandemic (European Parliament, 2020b, p. 48).

Respondents were asked to position themselves on a scale between two statements regarding the consequences of the restrictive measures in their country: comparing health benefits to economic damage (European Parliament, 2020b, pp. 16–18). Overall, respondents in two-thirds of the countries in the survey considered that health benefits were greater than economic damage, whereas respondents in six countries – Bulgaria, Hungary, Slovenia, Poland, Czechia and Italy – thought that economic damage was greater than the health benefits. Belgian respondents were equally split between the two views.

As countries emerged from lockdown, the June and July 2020 editions of the Commission's Public Opinion Monitoring Unit's newsletter tracked changing attitudes towards government responses and trust in public institutions (European Parliament, 2020a). By 1 July, more than 60% of Czech, Italian and Romanian respondents were satisfied with their governments' actions during the COVID-19 crisis. In Italy more than 60% of respondents expressed a negative attitude towards the EU. Romanians distinguished between different levels of government: more than 60% of respondents were satisfied with the measures taken by local authorities and their presidents, compared to 46% for the government. In Poland, 42% of respondents thought that the PiS government was performing well. In Sweden, confidence in the country's management of COVID-19 had fallen by 11 points to

45% since April, and satisfaction with the centre-left government's actions fell from 67% in May to 38% by 1 July. The newsletter reported findings from a study published by the Globsec think tank based in Bratislava showing that, in Slovakia, Lithuania, Latvia and Bulgaria, less than 50% of respondents backed 'liberal democracy with regular elections and multiparty system' as the best form of government.

Support for, and trust in, national leadership in managing the pandemic had reached over 80% in Austria and Cyprus, over 70% in Germany, Ireland, and Poland, over 60% in Greece, Hungary and Lithuania, and over 50% in Belgium and Italy, although Belgian respondents decried the fact that the country had frequently changed its health ministers. In France, the president saw his rating increase but only to 33%, while his prime minister stood at 40%. Satisfaction ratings with their governments' handling of the pandemic were found to be closely linked to general levels of support for government (European Parliament, 2020b, pp. 43–4): Denmark, Ireland, Portugal, the Netherlands, Finland, Austria, Greece and Slovakia reported scores over 70%, whereas Hungary, Bulgaria, France, Poland and Spain all reported satisfaction ratings under 50%.

According to Reuters Institute/University of Oxford (Fletcher et al., 2020), trust in the government in the UK declined substantially between 10/14 April (67%) and 21/27 May (48%). Trust in news organisations had also fallen to below 50%. Trust in the National Health Service (NHS), despite its iconic status, had declined but to a lesser degree and still stood at 86%. Levels of trust in the government and scientists were found to dip following revelations about the infringement of rules by one of the scientists advising government on lockdown, and then by the prime minister's chief adviser, for infringing the lockdown rules that they had helped to create (Mathieson, 2020; Waterson, 2020).

Comparing the performance of governments and their administrations

Examples drawn from the COVID–DEM Infohub (2020) country reports by lawyers and the reports published by the Robert Schuman Foundation (2020), mostly written by political scientists and journalists, illustrate the extent to which expectations based on the Thijs et al. (2018) and Bertelmann (2019b) indicators relate to outcomes. None of the member states at the top of the rank orders for the two composite indicators – Denmark, Finland and Sweden – ranked high for lockdown readiness and the stringency of the measures applied (Tables 3.1, 3.2 and 4.1). Denmark came closest to matching the criteria for administrative performance and quality of democracy (Cedervall Lauta, 2020). Sweden, for administrative performance, and Finland, for quality of democracy, both fell short (Cameron & Jonsson-Cornell, 2020; Scheinin, 2020). Bulgaria, Romania and Hungary justified their positions at the bottom of the rank order for the composite indicators, clearly demonstrating the need for further administrative reform. Bulgaria was accused of 'following the autocratic playbook for a long while, … creating loopholes to exploit the COVID-19 crisis' (Vassileva, 2020). Poland's harsh management of the crisis reinforced its low rank for quality of democracy (Jaraczewski, 2020).

During the first wave of the pandemic, governments were experimenting with different forms of interventions, based on what they believed at the time to be the best available scientific evidence, their assessment of the public mood and their own capacities, competences and ambitions. When read in conjunction with indicators of the quality of democracy, administrative performance, reports on the capacity of countries to manage the crisis effectively and results from opinion surveys, other factors emerge which may help to explain their shifting approaches. Extra-scientific factors, such as the feasibility of implementing scientific advice, time pressure, socioeconomic, political and institutional considerations were inherent to the decision-making process. These factors also influenced the effective implementation of response measures. Arguably, while being evidence informed, decisions could rarely be purely evidence based, not least due to the novelty of the pandemic.

5 Contextualising the impact of the COVID-19 pandemic within the European Union

The wide-ranging evidence accumulated in this book contests the value of comparisons based on a single dimension of the pandemic in a small number of EU member states, or with other countries in the world, if the statistics fail to take account of context. By drawing together the contextual dimensions examined in each of the preceding chapters, this chapter identifies overlapping clusters of countries that share comparable input variables – socio-demographic and epidemiological risk factors and policy settings – with a view to uncovering similarities and differences in outcomes as measured by COVID-19 cases and deaths. Granular analysis captures the great diversity of possible explanatory factors concealed within any single set of statistics or within clusters of countries. It shows that many of the factors considered to explain outcomes in specific spatial and temporal circumstances do not necessarily have the same explanatory value elsewhere. The implication is that certain policy interventions would not readily be transferable to different policy settings, at international, national or local levels, without contextually informed adaptations.

Contextualising COVID-19 cases and deaths

The chapters in this book have explored the multiplicity of socio-demographic, epidemiological and policy settings in which COVID-19 was to reach pandemic proportions in Europe. Each chapter contributes cumulatively to evidence about the importance of taking account of contextual dimensions when seeking to explain how different countries and clusters of countries performed in response to the unprecedented challenges posed by the pandemic for democratic societies. This chapter reviews the changing situation during the period when Europe was the epicentre of the pandemic. It begins by examining the progression of the disease within Europe before exploring the factors influencing and containing its spread in different clusters of countries (Figure 5.1).

In most of the EU member states that were among the first to be affected by the outbreak of the pandemic, and where the numbers of COVID-19 cases and deaths were relatively high, initially only deaths in hospitals were counted. The numbers subsequently increased rapidly when deaths in the

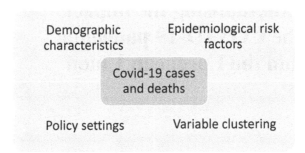

Figure 5.1 COVID-19 cases and deaths in context.

community, especially in care homes, were included, particularly in countries counting deaths where COVID-19 was the probable as well as the confirmed cause (Table 2.3).

Notwithstanding intractable issues of reliability and accuracy, statisticians used absolute figures for daily COVID-19 cases and deaths during the pandemic to monitor its progression and to inform policy decisions. A central tenet in this book is that, if international comparisons are to be meaningful, the statistics being compared need to be related to population size (per million inhabitants). Table 5.1 uses full dataset for the numbers of cumulative cases and deaths per million inhabitants for EU member states to illustrate the progression of the pandemic between 17 May (Table 2.2) and 17 July 2020, when the epicentre had moved from Europe to the Americas. By that time, only small numbers of new cases and deaths were being reported in the EU, although no member state recorded zero active cases, and new outbreaks were occurring in countries where the pandemic had largely been brought under control (Table 3.2).

Comparison of the death toll across the two dates shows that the four countries displaying the highest death rates per million inhabitants at 17 May retained their positions at 17 July 2020. The five countries with the smallest numbers of cases and deaths also retained their positions in the lower part of the table. The number of cases reported between the two dates increased most markedly in Sweden, Luxembourg and Portugal.

To overcome the limitations of cumulative daily counts, various attempts have been made to calculate the number of excess deaths during the pandemic's peak periods by comparing deaths from all causes for specific age groups with the same period in earlier years. Analysis of aggregate EuroMOMO (2020b) Z-scores (Table 2.4) showed that excess mortality rates were highest in Spain and England (over 40 points) for their peak weeks, followed by Belgium, France and the Netherlands (over 20 points). By 17 July (week 25), only Belgium, Spain and Sweden were displaying excess death rates greater than 2.

Calculations of excess mortality suggest that the full impact of the pandemic could be much greater than that in the published daily cumulative

Table 5.1 Cumulative cases and deaths per million inhabitants, 17 May and 17 July 2020

Cases 17 May		Cases 17 July		Death 17 May		Deaths 17 July	
Luxembourg	6291	Luxembourg	8438	Belgium	777	Belgium	845
Spain	5914	Sweden	7610	Spain	590	UK	664
Ireland	4877	Spain	6543	Italy	525	Spain	608
Belgium	4747	Belgium	5455	UK	508	Italy	579
Italy	3717	Ireland	5202	France	423	Sweden	554
UK	3540	Portugal	4685	Sweden	364	France	462
Sweden	2941	UK	4308	Netherlands	331	Netherlands	358
Portugal	2824	Italy	4032	Ireland	311	Ireland	354
France	2180	Netherlands	2997	Luxembourg	166	Luxembourg	177
Netherlands	2561	France	2663	Portugal	118	Portugal	165
Germany	2104	Germany	2409	Germany	96	Germany	109
Denmark	1875	Denmark	2265	Denmark	94	Denmark	105
Austria	1800	Austria	2139	Austria	70	Romania	102
Estonia	1334	Romania	1820	Romania	57	Austria	79
Malta	1237	Malta	1526	Finland	54	Hungary	62
Finland	1135	Estonia	1520	Slovenia	50	Finland	59
Romania	868	Finland	1316	Estonia	47	Slovenia	53
Czechia	790	Czechia	1271	Hungary	47	Estonia	52
Cyprus	758	Bulgaria	1173	Czechia	28	Bulgaria	42
Slovenia	705	Poland	1032	Poland	24	Poland	42
Lithuania	563	Croatia	984	Croatia	23	Czechia	33
Croatia	541	Slovenia	912	Lithuania	20	Croatia	29
Latvia	528	Cyprus	854	Bulgaria	16	Lithuania	29
Poland	482	Lithuania	699	Greece	16	Malta	20
Hungary	363	Latvia	625	Cyprus	14	Greece	19
Bulgaria	318	Hungary	443	Malta	14	Cyprus	16
Slovakia	273	Greece	378	Latvia	10	Latvia	16
Greece	270	Slovakia	357	Slovakia	5	Slovakia	5

Sources: Our World in Data (2020b, 2020c); Worldometer (n.d.b).

figures for COVID-19 deaths. Rough estimates for the EU member states reporting the highest cumulative deaths per million inhabitants (Table 2.5) show excess deaths for the duration of the pandemic to be 50% higher than expected in Spain, and around 40% higher in the UK, Italy and Belgium (Dale & Stylianou, 2020).

Throughout the period when the EU was the epicentre of the pandemic, Belgium remained the country with the highest death rates per million inhabitants, making it also the worst affected country in the world for this indicator. The high rate has been attributed to several factors. From the outset, Belgian authorities were including deaths in the community, especially in care homes, where it was reporting probable and confirmed deaths (Table 2.3), but this approach may only partially explain Belgium's persistently high daily mortality rate (Laborderie, 2020, p. 4). Many other factors need to be taken into account.

Demographic characteristics and COVID-19

Since the starting point for this study was to contest the validity of comparisons using absolute numbers of deaths in a small number of countries, Chapter 1 began by situating EU member states in relation to their socio-demographic characteristics focussing on population size and density. In Chapter 2, the patterning of death rates was considered in relation not only to population size and density but also to other geographical aspects of population distribution and social structure, with a view to identifying and explaining hotspots within countries. This section considers the combined impact of the various demographic factors that have been found to influence the course of the pandemic as it spread across EU member states (Figure 5.2).

Population size, density and urbanisation

Table 5.2 confirms that, as anticipated in Chapter 1, large population size is closely related to high death rates per million in the UK, Spain, Italy and France. This relationship is not found to apply in Germany and Poland, which display lower death rates in absolute and relative terms than might have been expected for their relatively large population size. Among the medium-sized countries, Belgium and Sweden report higher death rates than anticipated, whereas Romania, Greece, Czechia and Slovakia report relatively low death rates. The smallest countries, with below 5 million inhabitants, might be expected to display the lowest death rates, but Ireland and Luxembourg, Estonia and Slovenia report higher absolute and relative rates than anticipated for their population size.

The picture changes when death rates are considered in relation to population density. Here, Belgium and the Netherlands stand out as the countries with medium population size, but where high density is associated with high death rates, particularly in Belgium. The combination of large population size and high density in the UK and Italy also helps to explain their position among the countries displaying very high death rates, whereas the

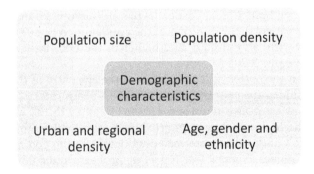

Figure 5.2 Demographic characteristics.

Table 5.2 COVID-19 deaths in relation to population size, density and urbanisation

Deaths 17 July		Population size		Density		Urbanisation	
Belgium	845	Germany	83.0	Malta	1548.3	Belgium	98.0
UK	664	France	67.0	Netherlands	504.0	Malta	94.6
Spain	608	UK	66.6	Belgium	375.3	Netherlands	91.5
Italy	579	Italy	60.4	UK	273.8	Luxembourg	91.0
Sweden	554	Spain	46.9	Luxembourg	235.1	Denmark	87.9
France	462	Poland	38.0	Germany	234.7	Sweden	87.4
Netherlands	358	Romania	19.4	Italy	202.9	Finland	85.4
Ireland	354	Netherlands	17.3	Denmark	138.0	UK	83.4
Luxembourg	177	Belgium	11.5	Czechia	137.7	France	80.4
Portugal	165	Greece	10.7	Poland	124.0	Spain	80.3
Germany	109	Czechia	10.6	Portugal	113.0	Greece	79.1
Denmark	105	Portugal	10.3	Slovakia	111.8	Germany	77.3
Romania	102	Sweden	10.2	Austria	107.1	Bulgaria	75.0
Austria	79	Hungary	9.8	Hungary	107.0	Czechia	73.8
Hungary	62	Austria	8.9	France	105.6	Hungary	71.3
Finland	59	Bulgaria	7.0	Slovenia	103.0	Italy	70.4
Slovenia	53	Denmark	5.8	Cyprus	94.4	Estonia	68.9
Estonia	52	Finland	5.5	Spain	93.1	Latvia	68.1
Bulgaria	42	Slovakia	5.5	Romania	84.0	Lithuania	67.7
Poland	42	Ireland	4.9	Greece	82.5	Cyprus	66.8
Czechia	33	Croatia	4.1	Croatia	73.2	Portugal	65.2
Croatia	29	Lithuania	2.8	Ireland	71.0	Ireland	63.2
Lithuania	29	Slovenia	2.1	Bulgaria	64.0	Poland	60.5
Malta	20	Latvia	1.9	Lithuania	44.7	Austria	58.3
Greece	19	Estonia	1.3	Latvia	30.4	Croatia	56.9
Cyprus	16	Cyprus	0.9	Estonia	30.4	Romania	54.0
Latvia	16	Luxembourg	0.6	Sweden	25.0	Slovenia	54.5
Slovakia	5	Malta	0.5	Finland	18.0	Slovakia	53.7

Sources: Eurostat (n.d.g): population density (km^2), 2018; Eurostat (n.d.h): population size (millions), 2019; United Nations (2018): urbanisation (% of territory).

same combination of demographic variables produces different outcomes in Germany and Poland for death rates. In France, large population size in combination with a lower ranking for density is associated with a relatively large number of deaths. The two smallest countries, Luxembourg and Malta, combine small population size with high density but with different outcomes: Luxembourg reports a much higher death rate than Malta. Denmark's relatively small size is accompanied by relatively high density and an intermediate position for COVID-19 deaths. The two medium-sized countries with the lowest densities, Finland and Sweden, also display different outcomes in terms of the numbers of deaths.

As the pandemic progressed, evidence became available enabling the identification of areas where hotspots were located and could be targeted by policy measures. As shown in Table 5.2, countries with persistently high death rates, the UK, Spain, Italy and France, display different levels of urbanisation, as defined with reference to agglomerations of more than 2,500 inhabitants. Belgium and the Netherlands, the two countries with the highest density overall, combine high COVID-19 death rates per million with very high rates of urbanisation. Several of the smaller countries with low death rates, Slovenia, Slovakia, Croatia, display low levels of urbanisation despite higher levels of overall density. Luxembourg and Ireland report similar death rates but different population sizes and urban densities. Despite their overall relatively low population density, Finland and Sweden display high rates of urbanisation due to the concentration of population in a small number of urban areas, but, as noted above, with very different death rates. Malta belies expectations: its death rate remains low despite its high urban density.

The impact of urbanisation is also determined by its regional spread. Analysis by Tallack et al. (2020) found that, in the UK excess death rates were greater than 30% in all its regions and nations. The authors attribute this patterning not only to the UK's greater overall population density but also to the greater dispersion of densely populated regions across the UK compared to Italy, Spain and France. London was initially the worst affected region in the UK. At the peak of the pandemic, excess deaths were more than 240% higher than usual, but subsequently other regions became hotspots. Aron & Muellbauer (2020) attribute the high and early peak in the UK to the London-centric location of the infection and the capital's international connectedness.

Similarities and differences were found in regional concentrations in other countries reporting high COVID-19 death rates. In Italy, for example, the pandemic peaked in Venetia and Lombardy, both wealthier regions in the north of the country, Lombardy because of its industry and international connectedness, and Venetia its tourism. Areas to the south, despite urban concentrations in Rome and Naples, were largely unaffected. In Spain, the virus spread most widely and rapidly in the more densely populated and prosperous urban agglomerations in Catalonia and the Madrid region. Madrid and Lombardy experienced earlier and higher peaks than London and were hit harder (Tallack et al., 2020).

Although France and Germany reported similar numbers of COVID-19 cases overall, France recorded almost twice the number of COVID-19 deaths (Deshaies, 2020b). In France, COVID-19 cases and deaths were highest in regions in the north and northeast and in the Paris area, whereas the centre, west and southwest were relatively unaffected. In Germany, the pandemic had spread across the border from Italy into Bavaria and Baden-Württemberg, and to a lesser degree to North Rhine-Westphalia. The northern and former East German states were relatively unaffected. Other disparities were observed within both countries. Munich, for example, reported a relatively low case fatality rate (the proportion of COVID-19 deaths, compared to the total number of cases diagnosed), whereas in France, the Vosges, in the northeast, reported ten times more COVID-19 deaths than the Haute-Vienne in the centre of France for an equivalent number of cases (Deshaies, 2020a). Despite their shared industrial history, the level of urbanisation and the daily interchange of frontier workers, differences were found in the spread of the virus between Alsace and Lorraine, in the northeast of France, and Saarland on the other side of the border in Germany.

Finland, the least densely populated member state, consistently reporting relatively low COVID-19 cases and deaths, is described as 'divided in two by the virus' (Petäistö, 2020, p. 19). The Helsinki metropolitan area accounted for three times more deaths than the rest of the country. In Estonia, a small, low-density country, the relatively higher number of cases and deaths was attributed primarily to an outbreak concentrated on the island of Saaremaa (ERR News, 2020). These comparisons confirm that the impact of urbanisation on the spread of the virus is not systematic or uniform across member states. Different combinations of demographic factors are needed to explain why ostensibly similar population sizes and densities produce different outcomes.

Age, gender and ethnicity

Readily accessible recent datasets are not available for age, gender and ethnicity variables across all member states. The few datasets that have been located provide clues as to why infection and death rates may be higher in some countries and regions than in others.

Compared to other epidemics, scientists have observed that older people are much more likely than younger age groups to die from COVID-19 (Petersen et al., 2020). In Chapter 1, old-age-dependency ratios (population aged over 65 in relation to total population) were found to be largest in Italy, Finland and Greece (Figure 1.1). EuroMOMO (2020b) indicators for excess deaths at different ages in 17 EU member states (Table 2.4) show that, in the peak weeks for the population aged over 75, Spain (over 40 points) reached the highest score, despite its relatively low position for old-age dependency. England (almost 30 points) was in second place, also with a relatively low old-age-dependency ratio, followed by Belgium and France (20 points). The Netherlands and Italy were lower down the score board. The two other countries with high dependency ratios, Finland and Greece, were even further down the table.

No complete datasets were available for all EU member states showing gender differences in the propensity to contract the virus and to die from it. Data collated by UN Global Health (2020) at 25 June 2020 suggest that women were more likely than men to contract the disease in all but six of the EU member states covered in the survey (Czechia, Greece, Latvia, Luxembourg, Portugal and Romania). Women were less likely than men to die from the virus except in Belgium, Estonia, Finland, Ireland and Slovenia. An analysis of the gender differential by age, carried out for the European

Commission in selected countries (Goujon et al., 2020, p. 5), also captured gender differences in positive COVID-19 cases. More cases were notified among men aged 55 to 80 years compared to women, while higher numbers of positive cases were reported among women aged 15–55 years and above 80. Across the seven countries analysed in detail – Italy, Belgium, Spain, Austria, the Netherlands, Germany and Portugal – Italy displayed the greatest propensity for men in the 55–80 age group to contract the disease compared to women. The difference was least marked in Portugal. Case fatality rates confirmed the male 'disadvantage', particularly for the age group 65–70.

Few EU member states collect information about COVID-19 deaths by ethnicity, generally for legal reasons. Where data are available for this variable, studies suggest that ethnic origins could be a contributing factor in explaining why some population groups were more likely to contract the disease and die from it. In the UK, for example, where the question has been most extensively studied, a review of inequalities in British society by the Institute for Fiscal Studies, an independent think tank, confirmed that some ethnic groups were being disproportionately affected by the pandemic (Platt & Warwick, 2020). They found that per capita COVID-19 hospital deaths were highest among the black Caribbean population, and three times those of the white British majority. Other minority groups, including Pakistanis and black Africans, were found to be recording similar numbers of hospital deaths per capita to the population average, while Bangladeshi fatalities were lower.

Data for deaths in France from all causes indicate that, during the pandemic, excess death rates among people born outside France increased by more than 50% among immigrants from the Maghreb (where most immigrants are born), by over 100% for those born in another African country, and over 90% from Asia-born immigrants, compared to 22% for French-born inhabitants (Papon & Robert-Bobée, 2020). Other studies suggest that higher rates of COVID-19 cases and deaths among ethnic minority groups are largely attributable to the risks associated with their relatively poor living and working conditions (Brandily et al., 2020).

Epidemiological risk factors and COVID-19

Public health covers all organised measures, whether public or private, at supranational, national or subnational levels, to prevent disease, promote health and prolong life for the whole population. The previous section demonstrated the value of situating comparisons in relation to the key demographic indicators examined in Chapter 1. The chapter also examined national health systems, public health capacity and health determinants in the expectation that, in combination with living and working conditions, they would contribute to, or mitigate, epidemiological risk factors (Figure 5.3).

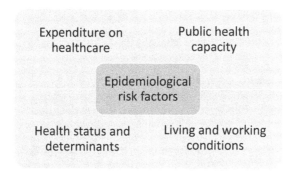

Figure 5.3 Epidemiological risk factors.

Expenditure on healthcare and public health capacity

Table 5.3 shows the relationship between healthcare expenditure in purchasing power standards (PPS), public health capacity and case fatality rates. Public health capacity is assessed by selected indicators for curative care beds in hospitals, preventable deaths per 100,000 inhabitants prior to the pandemic and by testing capacity at 17 July 2020.

At that time, France, the UK, Belgium, Italy, Hungary, the Netherlands and Spain were still reporting case fatality rates above 10%, whereas rates in Cyprus, Slovakia, Slovenia and Malta remained very low. The high rate in France was associated with relatively high spending on healthcare and low numbers of preventable deaths, but a low number of curative care beds in hospitals, in the period preceding the pandemic. The UK, Italy, Spain and Sweden ranked below France for per capita healthcare expenditure, although Italy, Spain and Sweden were performing relatively well in preventing premature deaths. Germany's high spending per capita and generous provision of curative care beds was not matched by a low preventable death rate or a very low case fatality rate. Nor are the low case fatality rates for Cyprus, Slovenia, Slovakia and Malta closely associated with any of the variables for healthcare capacity before the pandemic.

Although relatively high levels of unmet need were reported in some countries (Figure 1.4), few governments were prepared for the unprecedented demand during the pandemic. Information is not available across the EU about the supply of ventilators and personal protective equipment (PPE) in the early months of the pandemic, except to signal shortages. In Italy, the healthcare system in Lombardy was overwhelmed, which may have contributed to the spread of infection across hospitals and the large number of deaths among patients and staff (Charmelot, 2020, p. 27).

Data about testing capacity can be more easily accessed but is also subject to numerous caveats (Chapter 2, Table 2.2). The capacity to carry out diagnostic testing became widely considered as an important means of controlling the spread of the virus when associated with effective tracing and

Table 5.3 Per capita spending, curative care beds, preventable mortality, case fatality rates and testing

Per capita spending in PPS		Curative care beds per 100,000		Preventable deaths per 100,000		Tests per million 17 July 2020		Case fatality rate	
Germany	4.3	Bulgaria	617	Italy	175	Luxembourg	502830	France	17.3
Austria	3.9	Germany	602	Spain	182	Malta	248050	UK	15.4
Sweden	3.9	Lithuania	547	Cyprus	185	Denmark	222832	Belgium	15.4
Netherlands	3.8	Austria	545	Sweden	185	UK	186588	Italy	14.4
Denmark	3.7	Romania	525	France	191	Lithuania	175026	Hungary	13.9
France	3.6	Belgium	501	Netherlands	195	Cyprus	148771	Netherlands	12.0
Luxembourg	3.6	Slovakia	491	Luxembourg	204	Portugal	138644	Spain	10.9
Belgium	3.5	Poland	485	Ireland	205	Spain	128892	Sweden	7.3
Ireland	3.4	Hungary	427	Malta	207	Belgium	121890	Ireland	6.8
Finland	3.0	Slovenia	420	Belgium	220	Ireland	107704	Romania	5.6
UK	2.9	Czechia	411	Portugal	222	Italy	100955	Greece	4.9
Malta	2.7	Luxembourg	378	Denmark	230	Latvia	93201	Denmark	4.7
Italy	2.5	Greece	360	Austria	232	Estonia	85933	Germany	4.5
Spain	2.4	Croatia	351	Greece	236	Germany	82159	Finland	4.5
Czechia	2.1	Estonia	345	Finland	239	Austria	80628	Lithuania	4.2
Slovenia	2.1	Cyprus	340	Germany	241	Sweden	67494	Poland	4.1
Portugal	2.0	Latvia	330	UK	241	Slovenia	57426	Austria	3.7
Greece	1.7	Portugal	325	Slovenia	267	Czechia	57017	Bulgaria	3.6
Cyprus	1.7	Malta	318	Czechia	323	Finland	53220	Portugal	3.5
Slovakia	1.6	France	309	Poland	355	Poland	49838	Estonia	3.4
Lithuania	1.6	Netherlands	292	Croatia	370	Romania	47111	Croatia	3.0
Estonia	1.6	Finland	280	Estonia	385	Netherlands	44588	Latvia	2.6
Hungary	1.5	Ireland	277	Slovakia	417	Slovakia	43184	Czechia	2.6
Poland	1.4	Italy	263	Bulgaria	422	France	39868	Luxembourg	2.2
Croatia	1.3	Denmark	254	Lithuania	487	Greece	38227	Cyprus	1.8
Bulgaria	1.3	Spain	247	Hungary	506	Hungary	31343	Slovakia	1.4
Latvia	1.2	UK	211	Romania	512	Bulgaria	28287	Slovenia	1.4
Romania	1.0	Sweden	204	Latvia	521	Croatia	24224	Malta	1.3

Sources: Eurostat (n.d.j): treatable and preventable mortality (per 100,000 inhabitants); Eurostat (2020b, table 1): per capita spending (in PPS), 2017; Eurostat (2020e): curative care beds in hospitals (per 100,000 inhabitants) 2018; Our World in Data (2020a): case fatality rates; Worldometer (2020, n.d.b): tests per million 17 July 2020.

isolation. Table 2.2 included information about both absolute numbers of tests carried out and the numbers per million inhabitants for all EU member states at 17 May 2020. Table 5.3 shows relative positions for tests per million inhabitants at 17 July 2020. Data were not available at either date for all member states to show what proportion of the population was being tested. Comparison of the number of tests per million between countries would suggest that some of the smaller countries, Malta, Luxembourg, Lithuania and Cyprus, were probably testing larger proportions of their populations at both dates and doing so repeatedly. The Netherlands, Hungary, Croatia, Greece and Bulgaria consistently practised a low testing regime. Rates increased everywhere as testing capacity was built up, including in countries where it was already high. The UK moved furthest up the table as the government extended its testing regime. As in many other countries, priority continued to be given to essential workers and categories most at risk of contracting or transmitting the disease.

Luxembourg continued to be the country reporting the largest numbers of tests per million inhabitants, as well as the largest numbers of cases (Table 5.1). The substantial increase in the amount of testing in the UK between the two dates did not result in a change in its position for the number of confirmed cases. The countries reporting the smallest numbers of tests at both data points continued to report relatively low numbers of cases. These findings could mean that diagnostic testing does not capture mild or asymptomatic cases, and/or that relatively few new cases of infection were occurring or being reported. The doubling of the number of cases in Bulgaria, Poland and Romania between the two dates could be attributable to the increase in testing.

The case fatality rates displayed in Table 5.3 show that, with the exception of Hungary, the seven countries with rates over 10% were those reporting the highest death rates per million inhabitants at 17 July (Table 5.1). Conversely, the countries with low case fatality rates, with the exception of Luxembourg, reported some of the lowest death rates per million. The European Centre for Disease Prevention and Control (ECDC, 2020c, p. 9) cites a case fatality rate of over 25% for long-term care facilities across the EU. While Austria, Denmark and Germany managed largely to keep the virus out of care homes, governments in France, Italy, Spain, Sweden and the UK, which reported high overall case fatality rates, were criticised in the media for endangering the lives of people in residential care homes. The figures for case fatality rates should be interpreted with extra caution since most countries counted probable as well as confirmed COVID-19 deaths in care homes (Table 2.3). Older people in care homes were frequently suffering from life-threatening underlying conditions. The virus may not have been the main cause of mortality, although it may have brought forward death from other causes (Comas-Herrera et al., 2020).

In sum, countries with higher funding per capita and public health capacity, when associated with lower rates of infection, should, theoretically, have been in a better position to deliver a higher standard of care, thereby avoiding high mortality rates, achieving low case fatality rates and rapidly flattening the pandemic curve. The analysis in this section suggests that these epidemiological conditions may be necessary but are rarely sufficient to explain the full impact of COVID-19.

Health status and determinants

Since the chances of dying from COVID-19 are known to be higher for people with underlying health conditions, healthy life expectancy at age 65 provides an indication of the general health of a population. Table 5.4 shows the number of years that people (women and men) aged 65 could expect to live in good health before the outbreak of the pandemic. At age 65 people in Sweden, Malta, Ireland, Germany, Spain, Denmark and Belgium could expect to enjoy another 11 years or more of good health. By contrast, in

Table 5.4 Healthy life years at age 65, one-person households, diabetes in adults and obesity in adults

Healthy life at 65+		*1-person 65+*		*Diabetes adults %*		*Obesity adults %*	
Sweden	15.7	Bulgaria	20.1	Germany	15.3	Malta	28.9
Malta	14.3	Denmark	18.2	Portugal	14.2	UK	27.8
Ireland	12.9	Estonia	18.0	Malta	12.2	Hungary	26.4
Germany	11.9	Lithuania	17.6	Spain	10.5	Lithuania	26.3
Spain	11.4	Latvia	17.6	Cyprus	10.4	Czechia	26.0
Denmark	11.3	Finland	16.6	Czechia	10.2	Ireland	25.3
Belgium	11.1	Sweden	16.0	Austria	9.7	Bulgaria	25.0
France	10.8	Hungary	15.9	Hungary	9.3	Greece	24.9
UK	10.4	France	15.8	Finland	9.2	Croatia	24.4
Bulgaria	9.8	Romania	15.8	Slovakia	9.1	Spain	23.8
Netherlands	9.7	UK	15.0	Denmark	8.8	Latvia	23.6
Finland	9.5	Croatia	15.0	Romania	8.8	Poland	23.1
Italy	9.5	Germany	14.9	Bulgaria	8.3	Luxembourg	22.6
Luxembourg	9.1	Italy	14.9	Italy	8.3	Romania	22.5
Poland	8.5	Slovenia	14.6	Netherlands	8.1	Germany	22.3
Czechia	8.3	Czechia	14.5	Poland	8.1	Finland	22.2
Cyprus	7.5	Malta	14.4	Slovenia	7.8	Belgium	22.1
Austria	7.4	Belgium	13.9	France	7.6	Cyprus	21.8
Slovenia	7.4	Greece	13.6	Greece	7.4	France	21.6
Greece	7.3	Portugal	13.2	Latvia	7.4	Estonia	21.2
Portugal	7.3	Ireland	13.0	Sweden	7.2	Portugal	20.8
Hungary	7.2	Poland	13.0	Belgium	6.8	Sweden	20.6
Romania	6.1	Netherlands	12.6	Croatia	6.8	Slovakia	20.5
Lithuania	6.0	Austria	12.6	Luxembourg	6.5	Netherlands	20.4
Estonia	5.7	Spain	11.8	Estonia	6.2	Slovenia	20.2
Croatia	5.0	Slovakia	10.8	UK	5.6	Austria	20.1
Latvia	4.5	Luxembourg	9.9	Lithuania	5.4	Italy	19.9
Slovakia	4.4	Cyprus	6.5	Ireland	4.4	Denmark	19.7

Sources: Eurostat (n.d.e) : healthy life years; Eurostat (2017): elderly persons living alone at 65 and over, 2017; Statista (2020): diabetes in adults (in %), 2019; World Population Review (2020): obesity in adults (in %), 2020.

Romania, Lithuania, Estonia, Croatia, Latvia and Slovakia, healthy life expectancy was below 6.1 years. The implication is that fewer people in the last group of countries were likely to live to the age of 80, the age above which they would have been most likely to die if they contracted the disease.

The main underlying conditions associated with high COVID-19 death rates (comorbidities) are known to be diabetes, hypertension, chronic lung disease and cardiovascular disease. Rates are shown in Table 5.4 for the prevalence of diabetes and obesity for the adult population aged 20–79 years in EU member states in 2019/2020. In Germany, the highest prevalence of diabetes in 2019 was associated with the highest number of diabetes-related deaths per 1,000 (Statista, 2020). Patients who are diabetic and/or obese have been found to be particularly vulnerable to complications if they contract the virus (Diabetes UK, 2020; World Obesity, 2020).

Recent studies provide evidence indicating that low-income groups are at greater risk of being infected not only due to their overcrowded living conditions, as noted above for ethnic minority groups. They are also likely to be in poorly paid public office jobs in the service sector, especially health and social care, as well as in retailing and home deliveries, hospitality, entertainment and public transport, which were most affected by lockdown, loss of income and insecurity. These factors combine with the high prevalence of obesity, diabetes and heart conditions associated with poor outcomes (Marmot et al., 2020). In the UK, for example, data from the Office for National Statistics on age-corrected mortality rates by location confirm much higher COVID-19-related death rates in crowded living conditions in areas with the greatest economic deprivation (Aron & Muellbauer, 2020; Platt & Warwick, 2020; Tallack et al., 2020). Similar findings have been reported in France (Brandily et al., 2020).

Analysis in Chapter 1 suggested that household size and composition (Figure 1.8) might be important factors determining exposure to COVID-19. Table 5.4 shows the proportion of older people living alone. If they are in good health and able to self-isolate, as in the Nordic and Baltic states, where intergenerational coresidence is unusual, older people living alone might be expected to be less exposed to the risk of contracting the disease. If they are in poor health and dependent on help and support from non-resident family or community carers, as in Bulgaria, Latvia and Lithuania, they are more likely to be exposed to the disease and to the psychological problems resulting from self-isolation. Where intergenerational coresidence and support are common living arrangements, as Italy and Spain, and in countries where multi-person households are associated with overcrowding in densely populated urban areas, the risk of contracting the disease from younger generations and dying from it is likely to be much greater. Research (Ehl et al., 2020) has suggested that the differences in transmission rates from relations between France and Spain, where COVID-19 death rates are similar, may be attributable to traditionally higher levels of intergenerational coresidence in Spain. Measures to prevent primary infections among older people relying on physical distancing might, therefore, be more effective in countries with small households and more limited intergenerational coresidence.

Policy settings and COVID-19

Chapter 3 showed how governments in EU member states intervened to contain or eliminate the virus. Chapter 4 illustrated how knowledge about policy environments and administrative cultures contributes to an understanding of the performance of national governments and EU institutions as they dealt with COVID-19 and prepared for future pandemics.

Many difficulties were encountered in collating precise, reliable and comparable information about the relationship between policy settings and the impact of COVID-19 in EU member states. Problems arise not only owing to the lack of consistent data about the timing of the onset of COVID-19 and its peaks, but also because of variations in the speed and intensity with which measures were put in place and the severity of their application. Some EU member states made recommendations and issued advice, others introduced restrictive measures progressively and enforced them more or less stringently, while yet others declared an emergency and imposed draconian lockdown with penalties for non-compliance (Chapter 4). In many countries, the introduction of restrictive measures was found to be less controversial than decisions about lifting or easing lockdown, as governments, ministers of finance and health struggled with conflicting interests, pressures and advice and adapted their strategies, as well as their modes of governance, to prevent and contain new outbreaks.

In the years preceding the pandemic, Thijs et al. (2018) and the Bertelmann Stiftung (2019b) constructed composite indicators for public administration capacity and performance, and for quality of democracy (Chapter 4). They identified Sweden, Finland and Denmark as the countries that might be most effective in managing the pandemic. Their findings suggested that, in Hungary, Romania, Bulgaria, Greece and Croatia, governments were likely to be less well prepared administratively to confront the outbreak (Table 4.1). France, Malta, the Netherlands and Poland displayed much lower rankings for democratic indicators than for administrative capacity. Germany, Greece, Latvia, Lithuania, Portugal and Slovenia were higher in the rank order for democracy than for administrative capacity.

None of the countries at the top of the governance rankings for the two composite indicators displayed high rankings for lockdown readiness or stringency of measures applied when the pandemic was at its peak. Denmark moved up the rankings for stringency in July (Table 3.2), and it was the only one of the three countries at the top of the rank order for public satisfaction with the measures taken during the pandemic (Table 4.3). Denmark was joined by Finland among the countries that placed more trust in their governments than in scientists for information about the pandemic. In terms of outcomes, Sweden was among the countries displaying some of the highest figures for cases and deaths per million inhabitants, whereas Denmark and Finland maintained consistently lower positions in the rank order (Table 5.1).

All of the five countries with the lowest scores for governance indicators were in the medium range for speed of lockdown (Table 3.1). Bulgaria's and Hungary's relative positions increased for stringency of measures (Table 3.2). Croatia moved from being one of the countries with the most stringent measures to a position much lower in the rank order. Greece and Romania were positioned among the countries with medium rankings. Greece remained at the bottom of the rank order for cases and deaths throughout the pandemic, and Croatia was also among the lowest ranks (Table 5.1). Bulgaria saw its position move up the rank order, whereas Hungary was ranked lower for cases than for deaths. Croatians and Greeks were reasonably satisfied with their governments' performance during the pandemic, whereas Bulgarians, Hungarians and Romanians were least satisfied (Table 4.3). In none of the five countries did the public trust their government to provide reliable information about the pandemic, and in no country did the public place the EU among its three most trusted sources of information about the pandemic.

Analysis by lawyers of the legislative frameworks within which countries were operating during the pandemic highlighted the unevenness of responses across democracies as well as the challenges to their constitutional provisions. The boxes in Chapter 4 illustrated the diversity of legal instruments in each country, the changing distribution of legislative and executive powers, the shared responsibility for public health between central and regional governments, the legality of the measures implemented and the legal challenges faced by governments. In different combinations, these factors were found to affect the speed of their responses, the proportionality of the measures implemented and the outcomes in terms of COVID-19 cases and deaths.

Variable clustering during the pandemic

The great diversity of inputs and outputs made the task of comparing and contrasting the impact of the COVID-19 pandemic across the EU extremely complicated, since it was rarely possible to compare like with like, even over a small number of variables. The challenge of comparing dissimilar countries was already considerable without the additional problems of locating reliable and comparable datasets for all 27 EU members states and the UK, which was still included in most of the statistics for the European Economic Area if not for the EU. Scrutiny of compilations of datasets for EU member states tracking COVID-19 infections, deaths and testing illustrates how the positioning of different countries in frequently cited league tables varies depending, among others factors, on which countries are selected, how the data have been collected, reported and presented and, importantly, whether absolute or relative figures for tests, cases and deaths are being compared. This section examines different clusters or subsets of countries that have been found to share common features in their approach to the pandemic to determine whether they share similar outcomes.

Waves of EU membership

When clustered according to the timing of their membership of the EU (Figure 1.9 and Table 4.1), each wave of new members is found to display different combinations of socio-demographic, epidemiological and political traditions. Countries were constantly changing their governments, internal structures and even population size, as the two Germanys were united, and internal and external migratory movements contributed to population growth and change. The original member states represented – and continue to represent – a broad spectrum of countries in terms of socio-demographic characteristics, public health indicators, political systems and COVID-19 outcomes. The new wave of membership in 1973 brought three countries sharing a different conception of social welfare from the founder members. In the third wave, the other three Southern European member states joined Italy with their legacy of autocratic regimes. The fourth wave further reinforced the social-democratic model of welfare, while wave five added eight Central and Eastern European countries with their shared experience of Soviet rule, as well as the two small island states, each with their own chequered histories and traditions. The final wave brought three more countries from Eastern Europe, where reform of their judicial systems remained to be completed.

After more than six decades, the longstanding divisions between the founding member states in their approach to social policy resurfaced during the pandemic (Hantrais, 2019, 2020a). Germany, the largest and wealthiest of the six original EU member state, is often cited as a country that was able to avoid the worst impact of the pandemic. In comparison to the other large member states in the first wave (France and Italy), Germany had the advantage of a well-resourced health system and the capacity needed to manufacture and stock large quantities of medical and protective equipment. The country unilaterally closed its borders with its neighbours, and temporarily imposed export bans on medical supplies (Hamann, 2020). It introduced early large-scale testing and contact tracing (Aron & Muellbauer, 2020). German federalism allowed the most severely affected regions, Bavaria and Saarland, to implement strict measures to contain the spread of the virus, while the Chancellor, Angela Merkel, exercised strong leadership. She appealed to citizens to comply with the measures imposed to protect the whole population, resulting in a high level of satisfaction with her management of the pandemic.

France, by contrast, as a unitary bureaucratic country, with its less well-resourced public health system, was able to implement nation-wide decisions rapidly, but with the disadvantage that the government did not focus on hotspots and was less able to control the pandemic than Germany. Italy, the other large member state in this grouping, reached an early peak concentrated in its wealthier northern regions, resulting in one of the highest excess death rates, and incurring strong criticism of the government's response (Beqiraj, 2020; Charmelot, 2020). Belgium, which had a similarly high population size and density to the Netherlands, reported a much higher death rate per million, owing largely to the combination of political instability, the inability to coordinate its federal states and its problematic approach to reporting COVID-19 cases and deaths (Ganty, 2020; Laborderie, 2020). Luxembourg presented a different configuration from other founding member states. As one of the smallest but most densely populated and highly urbanised countries, with the lowest old-age-dependency ratio, a well-funded healthcare system and relatively high ratings for public administration, it reported the largest number of tests and cases but relatively low death rates. The government's response was criticised for its lack of clarity and direction (Stoppioni, 2020)

Herd immunity and frugality

A herd immunity or mitigation strategy, whereby a few countries introduced measures relying on voluntary compliance, is often contrasted with a more aggressive suppression strategy based on the implementation of a wide range of stringent measures, extending to limits on civil rights and liberties. Countries from the different waves of EU membership shifted between the two approaches, as their governments responded to the evolving pandemic.

When Europe became the epicentre of the pandemic, a few countries, the Netherlands, Sweden and the UK, deliberatively followed a herd immunity strategy in the expectation that transmission rates would be kept low if sufficient proportions of their populations were allowed to become immune to the disease. In a national address on 16 March, the Dutch prime minister, Mark Rutte, announced that his country would not go into complete lockdown (Cohen, 2020). Instead the aim was to develop immunity by letting large numbers of people contract the illness at a controlled pace, while protecting vulnerable groups. Rather than opting for a national lockdown, with potentially negative consequences and uncertain benefits, the Dutch government attempted to build herd immunity gradually by implementing an 'intelligent lockdown'. The prime minister acted as 'explainer-in-chief', and the government issued advice rather than orders (Buyse & de Lange, 2020). They left open the option of introducing additional measures later depending on how the virus developed. As the severity of the pandemic increased, and the government's approach began to be questioned, city mayors were authorised to issue and enforce emergency regulations, and to impose fines for non-compliance.

Like the Netherlands, the UK initially adopted a herd immunity strategy. Based on scientific advice, the UK government sought to balance 'the legitimate aim of protecting public health against the protection of civil liberties' (Grogan, 2020a). Policymakers followed rather than led public behaviour, only to find that they were accused of being responsible for more COVID-19 deaths because they had not acted more quickly and decisively (Aron & Muellbauer, 2020). The approach adopted, despite disagreement between scientists and policy advisers, was based on the expectation that public compliance with a full lockdown would be difficult to achieve if maintained for a long period of time. As public opinion shifted, and the politicians appeared to be losing the initiative, between 12 and 16 March tactics changed (Freedman, 2020). By July, the UK was the country with the highest ranking for the stringency of its lockdown measures and was near the top of the rank order for its testing capacity.

Sweden's measures in response to COVID-19 have been reported internationally as exemplifying a preferable alternative to highly restrictive measures (Grogan, 2020b). In the absence of a vaccine, the Swedish government sought to achieve herd immunity by allowing a sufficient proportion of the population to be exposed to, and infected by, the virus. The government did not introduce strict bans on travel and public events and gatherings, or school closures. Like the Netherlands and the UK initially, they issued non-binding recommendations. The government's decision not to take more drastic legal measures has been explained partly by doubts about the legality of such measures under existing delegations of power (Cameron & Jonsson-Cornell, 2020). The advice from the Public Health Authority was that most people could be relied upon to follow recommendations. The government enjoyed a high level of social trust and, in return, the public complied, at least in the early stages of the pandemic, and the damage to the economy appeared to be less severe than elsewhere in the EU. The country was expected to reach herd immunity during May, but by July, with older people accounting for more than 85% of the rapidly growing COVID-19 death toll, the Swedish approach was being called into question (Mock, 2020).

These three countries had in common with Denmark their concern to involve civil society by enabling citizens to take the initiative at local level before introducing legal requirements to bring about changes in behaviour. As a small country with a relatively homogeneous population, without adopting a herd strategy, Denmark managed to combine 'extraordinary law making, and (lawful) suspension of individual rights' (Cedervall Lauta, 2020). Executive power was increased while maintaining deaths at a level below that in the other three countries and without losing public support.

Denmark, the Netherlands and Sweden, which would have been joined by the UK had it remained in the EU, shared not only their concern to involve civil society in the decision-making process and to invoke the democratic concept of social responsibility. They also had in common that, with

Austria they belonged to what came to be known as the 'frugal four'. They were all net contributors to the EU's budget. Together, they rejected the initial Franco–German proposal for a grant-based EU recovery fund involving borrowing on capital markets on an unprecedented scale. Having been identified as one of the countries responsible for the spread of COVID-19, Austria differed from the herd immunity countries in that, under pressure from public opinion, the government adopted aggressive and early control strategies when a Tyrolean ski resort was identified as a major hotspot for spreading the virus across Europe (Lachmayer, 2020). The government's 'common sense' approach was designed to contain the spread of the virus and avoid overburdening the health system (Sauer, 2020). As a result, the number of cases and deaths remained low, and public satisfaction with the government's handling of the pandemic was high.

Ireland also came close to adopting a herd immunity strategy. Like the UK, Ireland is not a member of Schengen, and it did not close its borders at the onset of the pandemic. Nor did the government initially introduce strict lockdown measures. Ireland managed to avoid resorting to emergency powers by stretching the meaning of the constitution (Greene, 2020). In relation to size and density, Ireland displayed higher death rates than might have been expected (Table 5.2). As a net contributor to the EU budget, by not joining the frugal four, Ireland lost the opportunity to obtain a rebate in the budget negotiations (McGuirk, 2020).

Southern and Eastern cohesion

The 17 countries belonging to the 'friends of cohesion' group (essentially the Southern and Central and Eastern European member states) formed another cluster in their response to the EU's plans for supporting the economic recovery. In the EU budget negotiations, they were looking for reassurances that they would not be left on the periphery. Italy and Spain were aggrieved at not being supported by their European neighbours as they struggled to cope at the peak of the pandemic. Their leaders reiterated the importance of continuing support for cohesion policy if the EU was to meet its aim of achieving greater economic and social convergence among member states. Portugal remained in the higher ranks of countries for COVID-19 cases but ranked lower for deaths. The Portuguese government adopted a cautious approach during the early stages of lockdown, stating that 'no restrictions to freedom of expression and freedom of the press would be allowed during the crisis' (Violante & Lanceiro, 2020). Greece distinguished itself from France, Italy and Spain by remaining among the countries with the lowest rates for COVID-19 deaths. It displayed low rankings for administrative performance, democratic governance and health policy indicators, but a relatively high level of public satisfaction with government (Karavokyris, 2020).

Within the friends of cohesion group, Czechia, Hungary, Poland, Slovakia, the four Central and East European countries, previously known as the Visegrád Group, adopted a 'semi-frugal' position in the 2021–27 European budget discussions. They had been less affected by COVID-19 than the southern European member states (Table 2.1). They did not want to jeopardise their cohesion status and access to EU funds, since their economies had been severely affected by their early and stringent lockdown. Their populations retained the ingrained discipline acquired from living for a long period under Soviet rule. During the migration crisis in 2015, they had gained a reputation as nationalistic players, and as unconstructive and obstructive members of the EU, even though the political differences between them were growing and would be exacerbated by the COVID-19 crisis (Ehl, 2020). Hungary and Poland moved closer to becoming autocratic states and, like Italy, had turned to China to obtain supplies of ventilators and PPE when the EU failed to provide them (Macek, 2020).

Although the sixth wave countries, Bulgaria, Croatia and Romania, were ill-prepared to deal with the pandemic, they managed to contain the spread of the virus by introducing stringent anticipatory lockdown measures. Their approach presented significant constitutional challenges, particularly in Bulgaria and Romania, reflecting their low ratings for democratic indicators (Bačić Selanec, 2020; Selejan-Gutan, 2020: Vassileva, 2020).

Latvia, Lithuania and Estonia, which joined the EU at the same time as the Visegrád 4, formed a Baltic 'travel bubble' within the EU. They were relatively high in the table for democratic governance and administrative performance, and they introduced lockdown measures at an early stage. They were among the leaders in testing and suffered a relatively small number of deaths, without needing to overstep democratic controls (Dagilytė et al., 2020; Dimitrovs, 2020; Maruste, 2020).

The value of contextualising variables

This analysis of how combinations of variables contribute to outcomes shows that some countries belong to overlapping clusters while others are anomalous. Similarities and differences are found within each cluster, whether it be in terms of demographic, epidemiological or political characteristics, demonstrating the importance for comparative purposes of identifying the contexts within which variables are located and how they are conceptualised (Hantrais, 2009, pp. 74–6). When long-distance (all member states) and close-up (selected countries) perspectives are combined, the great diversity of the range of possible explanatory variables confirms the interest of adopting a 'variable distance' (Simmel, 1917).

A close-up or granular comparison of outcomes during the COVID-19 pandemic reveals differences that may not be apparent when aggregated national-level data are being compared from a long distance. It captures the great diversity of possible explanatory factors and the complexity of

EU-wide comparisons that is hidden within any single set of statistics. The implications of changing the mix or number of countries and the level of analysis affect both the findings and their interpretation.

In its guidance for social distancing measures, issued on 23 March 2020, aimed at minimising the spread of COVID-19, the ECDC (2020a) considered the generic challenges that EU governments would face in implementing appropriate measures, due not least to their different social, political and constitutional contexts, meaning that:

> What may be acceptable and feasible in one setting may not be in another. Societal norms and values underpinning freedom of movement and travel [for example] will need to be weighed against precautionary principles and the public acceptance of risks. It is important to consider, anticipate and plan for mitigation, while keeping in mind the considerable public reaction that social distancing measures [among others] may cause. There is no one-size-fits-all approach for implementation of social distancing measures.
>
> (ECDC, 2020a, p. 5)

The same conclusion could be applied to the multiplicity of factors explored in the present study.

Postface

The primary aim in this book was to alert the producers and users of the vast quantities of statistics tracking the progression of the pandemic across Europe to the dangers of making superficial comparisons whenever they sought to identify which countries were performing best or worst (Gibney, 2020). Another important objective was to explore lessons that decision-makers might draw from their own countries' experiences of the pandemic and those of other EU member states in preparation for subsequent outbreaks of the virus.

Knowledge about the disease, its treatments and how to prevent and control future surges is growing all the time. New knowledge changes preconceptions and assumptions, as well as the advice proffered by politicians and scientists. The unprecedented situation created by the pandemic prompted governments to introduce and enforce measures that would not have been publicly acceptable without the crisis. Their actions raised issues about how to safeguard the democratic principles that national governments agreed to observe as a condition of EU membership, by ensuring that greater central control over everyday life does not become the new normal. Another aspect of the new normal, which was set to outlive the crisis, was the accelerated and unprecedented development and adoption of technological solutions in response to the threats posed to economic and social life (Accenture, 2020).

Changes in patterns of work, education, entertainment and modes of delivery of healthcare and other public and private services during the pandemic created new opportunities and the need for innovative coping strategies. But these changes also intensified pressures on families, businesses and public institutions while exacerbating deep-seated socio-economic divides.

Policy learning from contextualised European comparisons

The contextualised comparisons conducted in this book reveal the great variety of factors that need to be considered if policy interventions are to achieve their objectives of eradicating the disease and supporting economic recovery. Arguably, lessons can be drawn from analysing the many possible reasons why certain measures appear to have been effective at a specific point in time in some places compared to others. In addition, lessons may be learnt from examining how policy responses, many of which were politically motivated and conflicted with scientific evidence, might need to be moderated and adapted if they are to be applied in different policy settings both within and across countries.

Throughout the book, analysis across European societies was hampered not only by the lack of full datasets for all EU member states but also by the variable quality of the available data and differences in data collection methodologies. Despite the best efforts of national and international statistical agencies and the many caveats they have issued, problems with data validity, reliability, consistency and accuracy mean that comparative analysis within and between countries can be a hazardous endeavour. A preliminary lesson to be drawn from this book is that, if international comparisons are to be meaningful, better data are needed to support fine-grain contextualised analysis.

A second lesson is that the countries selected for comparison should be matched on some key characteristics that may assist analysts in understanding why a particular combination of factors contributed to the observed outcome. At the point when the European epidemic was just past its peak, from a lawyer's perspective, Grogan (2020b) identified 'high levels of transparency in the decision-making process' as a common factor among what she assessed as 'successful states in epidemiological terms'. Public trust in the actions taken by governments was attributed to 'a co-ordinated effort of diverse and relevant expertise'. The public were more likely to accept and rally behind governments where the rule-of-law was seen to underpin interventions in terms of clarity, certainty, accessibility and congruence, and where the measures applied were in harmony with notions of social responsibility. Our analysis of EU member states suggests that the factors selected by Grogan undoubtedly contributed to public support for, and compliance with, government interventions in democratic states in the EU during the early stages of the pandemic, resulting in public satisfaction with the management and control of the pandemic. These factors were not, however, found to be sufficient, or even necessary, reasons for positive outcomes measured by the numbers of cases and deaths, since governments wavered, and public attitudes fluctuated, as priorities shifted between safeguarding public health and managing economic recovery.

Decision-takers, whatever their political persuasion, had understood the importance of rapidly identifying hotspots within countries or regions and of implementing efficient and effective targeted testing and tracing regimes without infringing privacy rules. They recognised the need for circumscribed travel bans and lockdown measures, implemented in cooperation with local authorities, if they were to limit the economic damage resulting from national lockdown. Most governments realised that they were more likely to be successful in containing the spread of the virus if they imposed proportionate, legally justified measures, if they targeted the necessary resources at the affected areas, and if their interventions were supported by the public.

A further take-away for governments is that the COVID-19 crisis acted as a trigger forcing them to innovate in ways that would otherwise have been inconceivable. The pandemic gave them license to use emergency powers to introduce changes in the way people live, work, use their leisure and are cared for, without going through the lengthy processes of democratic debate, consultation and scrutiny. Technological innovations that would have taken years to develop were scaled up within a matter of weeks, often at the price of accepting state surveillance and the infringement of individual autonomy and privacy. European comparisons suggest that citizens in the more authoritarian states were acquiescent when faced with emergency legislation and harsh restrictions on personal freedom as the price to pay for averting irreparable damage to their economies. Questions remain for both EU member states and other countries seeking to learn from them. Should big government be allowed to become a permanent feature of the new normal? Will governments learn from the crisis and use the opportunity to undertake the radical system change needed to achieve more equal and climate-friendly societies?

COVID-19 and EU social union

The sharing of competences for public health between EU institutions and member states, and within them between different levels of governance, was a further factor complicating the analysis in this book. Chapters 3 and 4 demonstrated how the European Commission tested the limits of its competence in the public policy field, and how it responded to challenges to its authority from member states. In seeking to carry out its treaty commitment for coordinating action across the EU and promoting European solidarity, the Commission relaxed EU rules on state aid and suspended regulations on public procurement and deficits. The 2020 budget discussions exacerbated divisions between the frugal four and the friends of cohesion. The cohesion group emerged as net 'winners' in the financial compromise reached on 20 July 2020, leaving several countries less than satisfied with the outcome.

Rather than healing the divisions revealed during the 2008–09 financial crises, the 2015 refugee and migration crisis, and when the post-Brexit social agenda for Europe was launched in 2017 (European Economic and Social Committee, 2017), COVID-19 aggravated latent tensions, divisions and dilemmas not only between but also within EU member states. The pandemic raised the question of whether a common EU public health approach could have saved more lives, and it cast doubt on the capacity of the July budget settlement to deliver a speedy economic recovery across the EU. Despite the show of unity during the Brexit negotiations, and the statement by the president of the European Commission (2020, 15 April) that 'the strength of Europe lies in its social and economic balance', the prospect of achieving ever closer social union seemed to be on hold, at least for so long as 'Union action shall respect the responsibilities of the Member States for the definition of their health policy and for the organisation and delivery of health services and medical care' (Article 168, 2007 Lisbon Treaty).

References

Accenture (2020). COVID-19: Post-Coronavirus technology trends, *Technology Vision 2020*, 19 June 2020. https://www.accenture.com/us-en/insights/technology/tech-vision-coronavirus-trends

Adam, D. (2020). The limits of R: What the reproduction number can and can't tell us about managing COVID-19, *Nature, 583*, 346–8. https://media.nature.com/original/magazine-assets/d41586-020-02009-w/d41586-020-02009-w.pdf

Adonis, A. (2018). *Half in half out: Prime ministers on Europe*, London: Biteback. https://www.bitebackpublishing.com/books/half-in-half-out

Aget, A. (2020). La plupart des cas de COVID ne propagent pas le virus – ce sont juste les super-propagateurs que nous devons arrêter, *UP Magazine*, 15 June 2020. https://up-magazine.info/le-vivant/sciences/60318-la-plupart-des-cas-de-covid-ne-propagent-pas-le-virus-ce-sont-juste-les-super-propagateurs-que-nous-devons-arreter/

Alemanno, A. (2020). Testing the limits of EU health emergency power, *Verfassungsblog on matters constitutional*, 18 April 2020. https://verfassungsblog.de/testing-the-limits-of-eu-health-emergency-power/

Anderson, J. (2020). Sweden's very different approach to Covid-19, *Quartz*, 27 April 2020. https://qz.com/1842183/sweden-is-taking-a-very-different-approach-to-covid-19/

Ángel Presno Linera, M. (2020). Beyond the state of alarm: COVID-19 in Spain, *Verfassungsblog on matters constitutional*, 13 May 2020. https://verfassungsblog.de/beyond-the-state-of-alarm-covid-19-in-spain/

Aron, J. & Muellbauer, J. (2020). *Measuring excess mortality: The case of England during the Covid-19 pandemic*, INET Oxford Working Paper no. 2020-11. https://www.inet.ox.ac.uk/files/revised-15.54-18-May-20-Aron-Muellbauer-Revised-INET-Excess-Mortality-article-x.pdf

Bačić Selanec, N. (2020). Croatia's response to COVID-19: On legal form and constitutional safeguards in times of pandemic, *Verfassungsblog on matters constitutional*, 9 May 2020. https://verfassungsblog.de/croatias-response-to-covid-19-on-legal-form-and-constitutional-safeguards-in-times-of-pandemic/

Bayer, L. (2020). Brussels drops lockdown exit plan after anger from capitals, *Politico EU*, 7 April 2020. https://www.politico.eu/article/commission-to-unveil-exit-strategy-as-countries-push-to-lift-corona-measures/

Bayer, L. & Cokeleare, H. (2020). The EU travel ban explained: Governments force Commission into U-turn over fears it was moving too quickly, *Politico EU*, 17

March 2020. https://www.politico.eu/article/the-eu-european-union-coronavirus-covid19-travel-ban-explained/

BBC (2020). Coronavirus: The world in lockdown in maps and charts, *BBC News*, 7 April 2020. https://www.bbc.co.uk/news/world-52103747

Beqiraj, J. (2020). Italy's Coronavirus legislative response: Adjusting along the way, *Verfassungsblog on matters constitutional*, 8 April 2020. https://verfassungsblog.de/italys-coronavirus-legislative-response-adjusting-along-the-way/

Bertelmann Stiftung (2019a). Sustainable government indicators: Health policy, *SGI Network*. https://www.sgi-network.org/2019/Policy_Performance/Social_Policies/Health/Health_Policy

Bertelmann Stiftung (2019b). Sustainable government indicators: Quality of democracy, *SGI Network*. https://www.sgi-network.org/2019/Democracy/Quality_of_Democracy

Bischoff, W. (2020). Vitamin D, explaining R and the 2 metre rule, *More or less*, BBC Radio 4, 13 May 2020. https://www.bbc.co.uk/sounds/play/m000j2r7

Bodeux, L. & Gnes, D. (2020). Undocumented workers are COVID-19 'elephant in room', *EU Observer*, April 2020. https://www.business-humanrights.org/en/eu-urged-to-ensure-labour-and-health-protection-for-migrant-farm-workers-amid-covid-19-crisis

Brandily, P., Brebion, C., Briole, S. & Khoury, L. (2020). A poorly understood disease? The unequal distribution of excess mortality due to COVID-19 across French municipalities, MedRxis preprint, 10 July 2020. DOI: 10.1101/2020.07.09.20149955

Braw, E. (2020). Beware of bad Samaritans: China and Russia are sending medical aid to Italy and other coronavirus-stricken countries, but their motives aren't so altruistic. *Foreign Policy News*, 30 March 2020. https://foreignpolicy.com/2020/03/30/russia-china-coronavirus-geopolitics/

Brzozowski, A. (2020). All you need to know about Europe lifting its internal border restrictions, *Euractiv*, 16 June 2020. https://www.euractiv.com/section/politics/news/all-you-need-to-know-about-europe-lifting-its-internal-border-restrictions/

Burn-Murdoch, J. (2020). Antibody tests, early lockdown advice and European deaths, *More or less*, BBC Radio 4, 10 June 2020. https://www.bbc.co.uk/sounds/play/m000jw02

Buyse, A. & de Lange, R. (2020). The Netherlands: Of rollercoasters and elephants, *Verfassungsblog on matters constitutional*, 8 May 2020. https://verfassungsblog.de/the-netherlands-of-rollercoasters-and-elephants/

Cameron, I. & Jonsson-Cornell, A. (2020). Sweden and COVID 19: A constitutional perspective, *Verfassungsblog on matters constitutional*, 7 May 2020. https://verfassungsblog.de/sweden-and-covid-19-a-constitutional-perspective/

Cedervall Lauta, K. (2020). Something is forgotten in the state of Denmark: Denmark's response to the COVID-19 pandemic, *Verfassungsblog on matters constitutional*, 4 May 2020. https://verfassungsblog.de/something-is-forgotten-in-the-state-of-denmark-denmarks-response-to-the-covid-19-pandemic/

Charmelot, J. (2020). Covid Italian style: The Lombardian case, in Robert Schuman Foundation (ed.), *Managing Covid-19, a journey through Europe*, 30 April 2020, pp. 27–9. https://www.robert-schuman.eu/en/doc/divers/Covid-19_Through_Europe.pdf

Chazan, G. (2020). Germany's *Länder* break ranks with Merkel to ease lockdown, *Financial Times*, 6 May 2020. https://www.ft.com/content/77535d00-b1ab-4066-88c0-6402cd17fd4f

Chu, D.K., Akl, E.A., Duda, S., Solo, K., Yaacoub, S. & Schünemann, H.J. (2020). Physical distancing, face masks, and eye protection to prevent person-to-person transmission of SARS-CoV-2 and COVID-19: A systematic review and meta-analysis, *Lancet*, *395*, 1973–97, online 1 June 2020. DOI: 10.1016/S0140-6736(20)31142-9

Ciminelli, G. & Silvia, G-M. (2020). COVID-19 in Italy: An analysis of death registry data, *Vox CEPR Policy Portal*, 22 April 2020. https://voxeu.org/article/covid-19-italy-analysis-death-registry-data

Cohen, J. (2020). Caught between herd immunity and national lockdown: The Netherlands hit hard by Covid-19 (update), *Forbes*, 27 March 2020. https://www.forbes.com/sites/joshuacohen/2020/03/27/caught-between-herd-immunity-and-national-lockdown-holland-hit-hard-by-covid-19/

Comas-Herrera, A., Zalakaín, J., Litwin, C., Hsu, A.T., Lane, N. & Fernández, J-L. (2020). *Mortality associated with COVID-19 outbreaks in care homes: Early international evidence*, International Long-Term Care Network, 3 May 2020. https://ltccovid.org/wp-content/uploads/2020/05/Mortality-associated-with-COVID-3-May-final-6.pdf

COVID–DEM Infohub (n.d.). *COVID–DEM*, COVID-DEM – dem-dec. https://www.democratic-decay.org/covid-dem

COVID–DEM Infohub (2020). List of country reports, COVID 19 and states of emergency, *Verfassungsblog on matters constitutional*, 6 April 2020. https://verfassungsblog.de/introduction-list-of-country-reports/

Dagilytė, E., Padskočimaitė, A. & Vainorienė, A. (2020). Lithuania's response to COVID-19: Quarantine through the prism of human rights and the rule of law, *Verfassungsblog on matters constitutional*, 14 May 2020. https://verfassungsblog.de/lithuanias-response-to-covid-19-quarantine-through-the-prism-of-human-rights-and-the-rule-of-law/

Dale, B. & Stylianou, N. (2020). Coronavirus: What is the true death toll of the pandemic? *BBC News*, 18 June 2020. https://www.bbc.co.uk/news/world-53073046

Daly, M., Ebbinghaus, B., Lehner, L., Naczyk, M. & Vlandas, T. (2020) *Tracking policy responses to COVID-19: Opportunities, challenges and solutions*, Oxford supertracker policy brief, 14 September 2020. https://supertracker.spi.ox.ac.uk/assets/STBrief-1.pdf

Daly, T.G. (2020). Democracy and the global emergency: Shared experiences, starkly uneven impacts, *Verfassungsblog on matters constitutional*, 15 May 2020. https://verfassungsblog.de/democracy-and-the-global-emergency-shared-experiences-starkly-uneven-impacts/

Deshaies, M. (2020a). Géographie de la mortalité due au Covid-19 en France et en Allemagne, *The Conversation*, 19 June 2020. https://theconversation.com/geographie-de-la-mortalite-due-au-covid-19-en-france-et-en-allemagne-141235

Deshaies, M. (2020b). Géographie de la pandémie de Covid-19 en France et en Allemagne: Premiers enseignements, *The Conversation*, 26 May 2020. https://theconversation.com/geographie-de-la-pandemie-de-covid-19-en-france-et-en-allemagne-premiers-enseignements-139367

Desvars-Larrive, A., Dervic, E., Niederkrotenthaler, T., Di Natale, A., Chen, J., Lasser, A. et al. (2020). A structured open dataset of government interventions in response to COVID-19, *Scientific Data*, *7*(1), 285. DOI: 10.1038/s41597-020-00609-9

Diabetes UK (2020). NHSE statistics on coronavirus deaths in people with diabetes, *Diabetes UK*, 25 May 2020. https://www.diabetes.org.uk/about_us/news/corona virus-statistics

Dimitrovs, A. (2020). COVID-19 in Latvia: Precaution above all, *Verfassungsblog on matters constitutional*, 2 May 2020. https://verfassungsblog.de/covid-19-in-latvia-precaution-above-all/

Donnelly, C. (2020). Mitigation or suppression: What's best to tackle coronavirus? *More or less*, BBC Radio 4, 25 April 2020. https://www.bbc.co.uk/programmes/w3csz3sg

Donovan, D. (2020). Global health map tracks coronavirus outbreak in near real time, *Coronavirus Information and Resources for JHU*, 23 January 2020. https://hub.jhu.edu/2020/01/23/coronavirus-outbreak-mapping-tool-649-em1-art1-dtd-health/

Ehl, M. (2020). The other frugal four: The V4 closely watches the EU budget discussion, *Visegrad Insight*, 27 May 2020. https://visegradinsight.eu/the-other-frugal-four-v4-eu-budget/

Ehl, M., Esteve, A., Permanyer, I., Boertien. D. & Vaupel, J.W. (2020). National age and coresidence patterns shape COVID-19 vulnerability, *Proceedings of the National Academy of Sciences of the United States of America*, 23 June 2020. DOI: 10.1073/pnas.2008764117

ERR News (2020). Timeline: How Saaremaa became the epicenter of Estonia's COVID-19 outbreak, 6 April 2020. https://news.err.ee/1073140/timeline-how-saaremaa-became-the-epicenter-of-estonia-s-covid-19-outbreak

Eurobarometer (2017). *Future of Europe: Social issues*, Special Eurobarometer Report 267, 17 November 2020. https://ec.europa.eu/commfrontoffice/publicopinion/index.cfm/ResultDoc/download/DocumentKy/80645

Eurobarometer (2019). *Standard Eurobarometer 92: First results*, December 2019. https://www.dnevnik.bg/file/4008585.pdf

EuroMOMO (2020a). EuroMOMO bulletin: Week 20, 2020, *EuroMOMO bulletins*. https://www.euromomo.eu/bulletins/2020-20

EuroMOMO (2020b). Excess mortality: Z-scores by country, *EuroMOMO graphs and maps*. https://www.euromomo.eu/graphs-and-maps

EuroMOMO (2020c). What is a Z-score? https://www.euromomo.eu/how-it-works/what-is-a-z-score/

European Centre for Disease Prevention and Control (ECDC) (2020a). *Considerations relating to social distancing measures in response to COVID-19*, second update, 23 March 2020. https://www.ecdc.europa.eu/sites/default/files/documents/covid-19-social-distancing-measuresg-guide-second-update.pdf

European Centre for Disease Prevention and Control (ECDC) (2020b). *Coronavirus disease 2019 (COVID-19) in the EU/EEA and the UK*, eighth update (Rapid risk assessment), 8 April 2020. https://www.ecdc.europa.eu/sites/default/files/documents/covid-19-rapid-risk-assessment-coronavirus-disease-2019-eighth-update-8-april-2020.pdf

European Centre for Disease Prevention and Control (ECDC) (2020c). *Coronavirus disease 2019 (COVID-19) in the EU/EEA and the UK*, tenth update (Rapid risk assessment), 11 June 2020. https://www.ecdc.europa.eu/sites/default/files/documents/RRA-COVID19-update10-2020-06-11.pdf

European Centre for Disease Prevention and Control (ECDC) (2020d). *Disease prevention and control, using face masks in the community*, Technical report, 8 April

2020. https://www.ecdc.europa.eu/sites/default/files/documents/COVID-19-use-face-masks-community.pdf

European Commission (n.d.a). Country health profiles, *State of health in the EU.* https://ec.europa.eu/health/state/country_profiles_en

European Commission (n.d.b). ECHI – European core health indicators, *Indicators and data.* https://ec.europa.eu/health/indicators/echi/list_en

European Commission (n.d.c). III Public support/Social protection and inclusion, *Social Scoreboard.* https://composite-indicators.jrc.ec.europa.eu/social-scoreboard/explorer?primarychart=table

European Commission (2017). *European Pillar of Social Rights – booklet*, no. 18, 16 November 2017. https://ec.europa.eu/commission/publications/european-pillar-social-rights-booklet_en

European Commission (2018). *Challenges in long-term care in Europe: A study of national policies*, European Social Policy Network (ESPN). https://ec.europa.eu/social/main.jsp?langId=en&catId=89&newsId=9185

European Commission (2020, 16 March). Communication from the Commission to the European Parliament, the European Council and the Council, COVID-19: Temporary restriction on non-essential travel to the EU, COM(2020) 115 final. https://ec.europa.eu/transparency/regdoc/rep/1/2020/EN/COM-2020-115-F1-EN-MAIN-PART-1.PDF

European Commission (2020, 18 March). EU recommendations for testing strategies. https://ec.europa.eu/info/sites/info/files/covid19_-_eu_recommendations_on_testing_strategies_v2.pdf

European Commission (2020, 19 March). COVID-19: Commission creates first ever rescEU stockpile of medical equipment, Press release. https://ec.europa.eu/commission/presscorner/detail/en/ip_20_476

European Commission (2020, 30 March). Communication from the Commission to the European Parliament, the European Council and the Council, COVID-19: Guidance on the implementation of the temporary restriction on non-essential travel to the EU, on the facilitation of transit arrangements for the repatriation of EU citizens, and on the effects on visa policy, C(2020) 2050 final. https://ec.europa.eu/home-affairs/sites/homeaffairs/files/what-we-do/policies/european-agenda-migration/20200330_c-2020-2050-report_en.pdf

European Commission (2020, 2 April). Proposal for a Council Regulation on the establishment of a European instrument for temporary support to mitigate unemployment risks in an emergency (SURE) following the COVID-19 outbreak, COM/2020/139 final. https://eur-lex.europa.eu/legal-content/EN/TXT/?uri=COM%3A2020%3A139%3AFIN

European Commission (2020, 8 April). Guidelines on the optimal and rational supply of medicines to avoid shortages during the COVID-19 outbreak, C(2020) 2272 final. https://ec.europa.eu/info/sites/info/files/communication-commission-guidelines-optimal-rational-supply-medicines-avoid.pdf

European Commission (2020, 15 April). Coronavirus: European roadmap shows path towards common lifting of containment measures, Press release. https://ec.europa.eu/commission/presscorner/detail/en/IP_20_652

European Commission (2020, 16 April). Joint European Roadmap towards lifting COVID-19 containment measures, 16 April 2020. https://ec.europa.eu/info/sites/info/files/communication_-_a_european_roadmap_to_lifting_coronavirus_containment_measures_0.pdf

European Commission (2020, 27 May). Communication from the Commission to the European Parliament, the European Council, the Council, the European Economic and Social Committee and the Committee of the Regions, Europe's moment: Repair and prepare for the next generation, COM(2020) 456 final. https://ec.europa.eu/info/sites/info/files/communication-europe-moment-repair-prepare-next-generation.pdf

European Council (2020a). Video conference of members of the European Council, 10 March 2020. https://www.consilium.europa.eu/en/meetings/european-council/2020/03/10/

European Council (2020b). Video conference of ministers of health, 15 April 2020. https://www.consilium.europa.eu/en/meetings/epsco/2020/04/15/

European Council/Council of the European Union (2020). Members of the European Council, June 2020. https://www.consilium.europa.eu/en/european-council/members/

European Economic and Social Committee (2017). *White paper on the future of Europe: National consultations of organized civil society*, May–June 2017. https://www.eesc.europa.eu/sites/default/files/resources/docs/white-paper-on-the-future-of-europe---compilation---en.pdf

European Parliament (2020a). Public opinion monitoring in the time of Covid-19, *Newsletters*, March–. https://www.europarl.europa.eu/at-your-service/en/be-heard/eurobarometer/public-opinion-in-the-time-of-covid-19

European Parliament (2020b). *Uncertainty/EU/hope public opinion in times of Covid-19*, Public Opinion Monitoring Unit, 3 June 2020. https://www.europarl.europa.eu/at-your-service/files/be-heard/eurobarometer/2020/public_opinion_in_the_eu_in_time_of_coronavirus_crisis/report/en-covid19-survey-report.pdf

European Union Aviation Safety Agency (EASA/ECDC, 2020). Covid-19 aviation health safety protocol, 21 May 2020. https://www.easa.europa.eu/document-library/general-publications/covid-19-aviation-health-safety-protocol

Eurostat (2017). *What is the share of the elderly who live alone? A look at the lives of the elderly in the EU today*, Eurostat infograph. https://ec.europa.eu/eurostat/cache/infographs/elderly/index.html

Eurostat (n.d.a). Curative care bed occupancy rate, 2018. https://appsso.eurostat.ec.europa.eu/nui/show.do?dataset=hlth_co_bedoc&lang=en

Eurostat (n.d.b). Distribution of households by household type from 2003 onwards – EU-SILC survey, 2018. https://appsso.eurostat.ec.europa.eu/nui/show.do?dataset=ilc_lvph02&lang=en

Eurostat (n.d.c). General government expenditure by function: Health, 2010, 2018. https://ec.europa.eu/eurostat/tgm/refreshTableAction.do;jsessionid=5HWsknLwHIT8nZvCggmNPfUhHEKbe4GWWk74kb_jsJwP-wOloU1N!-1353419636?tab=table&pcode=tepsr_sp110&language=en

Eurostat (n.d.d). Healthy life years at age 65 by sex (in years), 2018/2019. https://ec.europa.eu/eurostat/tgm/refreshTableAction.do?tab=table&plugin=1&pcode=tepsr_sp320&language=en

Eurostat (n.d.e). Old-age-dependency ratio, 2019. https://ec.europa.eu/eurostat/databrowser/view/tps00198/default/table?lang=en

Eurostat (n.d.f). Out-of-pocket expenditure on healthcare % share of total current health expenditure), 2018. https://ec.europa.eu/eurostat/tgm/table.do?tab=table&init=1&language=en&pcode=tepsr_sp310

Eurostat (n.d.g). Population density, 2018. https://ec.europa.eu/eurostat/databrowser/view/tps00003/default/table?lang=en

Eurostat (n.d.h). Population on 1 January 2019 by age and sex. https://appsso.eurostat.ec.europa.eu/nui/show.do?dataset=demo_pjan&lang=en

Eurostat (n.d.i). Practising physicians per 100,000 inhabitants, 2018. https://ec.europa.eu/eurostat/tgm/table.do?tab=table&init=1&language=en&pcode=tps00044&plugin=1

Eurostat (n.d.j). Self-reported unmet need for medical care by sex, 2018/2019. https://ec.europa.eu/eurostat/tgm/table.do?tab=table&init=1&language=en&pcode=tespm110

Eurostat (n.d.j). Treatable and preventable mortality of residents by cause and sex, 2017. https://appsso.eurostat.ec.europa.eu/nui/show.do?dataset=hlth_cd_apr&lang=en

Eurostat (2020a). Covid-19: Support for statisticians, *Your key to European statistics.* https://ec.europa.eu/eurostat/data/metadata/covid-19-support-for-statisticians

Eurostat (2020b). Healthcare expenditure statistics, *Statistics Explained.* https://ec.europa.eu/eurostat/statistics-explained/pdfscache/37773.pdf

Eurostat (2020c). Healthcare personnel statistics – nursing and caring professionals, *Statistics Explained.* https://ec.europa.eu/eurostat/statistics-explained/index.php/Healthcare_personnel_statistics_-_nursing_and_caring_professionals

Eurostat (2020d). Healthcare personnel statistics – physicians, *Statistics Explained.* https://ec.europa.eu/eurostat/statistics-explained/pdfscache/37382.pdf

Eurostat (2020e). Healthcare resource statistics – beds, *Statistics Explained.* https://ec.europa.eu/eurostat/statistics-explained/index.php/Healthcare_resource_statistics_-_beds

Eurydice (2020). How is Covid-19 affecting schools in Europe? 2 April 2020. https://eacea.ec.europa.eu/national-policies/eurydice/content/how-covid-19-affecting-schools-europe_en

Flaxman, S., Mishra, S., Gandy, A., Unwin, H., Coupland, H., Zhu, H. et al. (2020). *Estimating the number of infections and the impact of non-pharmaceutical interventions on COVID-19 in 11 European countries*, Imperial College COVID-19 Response Team, Report 13, 30 March 2020. DOI: 10.25561/77731

Fletcher, R., Kalogeropoulos, A. & Nielsen, R.K. (2020). Trust in UK government and news media: COVID-19 information down, concerns over misinformation from government and politicians up, *The UK COVID-19 news and information project*, fourth factsheet, 1 June 2020. https://reutersinstitute.politics.ox.ac.uk/trust-uk-government-and-news-media-covid-19-information-down-concerns-over-misinformation

Foote, N. (2020). Working conditions in meat processing plants make them hotbed for COVID-19, *Euractiv*, 26 June 2020. https://www.euractiv.com/section/agriculture-food/news/working-conditions-in-meat-processing-plants-make-them-hotbed-for-covid-19/

Freedman, L. (2020). Strategy for a pandemic: The UK and Covid-19, *Survival*, 62(3), 25–76. DOI: 10.1080/00396338.2020.1763610

Ganty, S. (2020). Belgium and COVID-19: When a health crisis replaces a political crisis, *Verfassungsblog on matters constitutional*, 21 April 2020. https://verfassungsblog.de/belgium-and-covid-19-when-a-health-crisis-replaces-a-political-crisis/

Gibney, E. (2020). Whose coronavirus strategy worked best? Scientists hunt most effective policies, *Nature, 581,* 15–16. https://media.nature.com/original/magazine-assets/d41586-020-01248-1/d41586-020-01248-1.pdf

Goujon, A., Natale, F., Ghio, D., Conte, A. & Dijkstra, L. (2020). *Age, gender, and territory of COVID-19 infections and fatalities,* JRC technical report, Luxembourg: Publications Office of the European Union. https://publications.jrc.ec.europa.eu/repository/bitstream/JRC120680/gender_territory_covid19_online.pdf

Greene, A. (2020). Ireland's response to the COVID-19 pandemic, *Verfassungsblog on matters constitutional,* 11 April 2020. https://verfassungsblog.de/irelands-response-to-the-covid-19-pandemic/

Grogan, J. (2020a). Right restriction or restricting rights? The UK acts to address COVID-19, *Verfassungsblog on matters constitutional,* 17 April 2020. https://verfassungsblog.de/right-restriction-or-restricting-rights-the-uk-acts-to-address-covid-19/

Grogan, J. (2020b). States of emergency, *Verfassungsblog on matters constitutional,* 26 May 2020. https://verfassungsblog.de/states-of-emergency/

Hale, T., Phillips, T., Petherick, A., Kira, B., Angrist, N., Aymar, K. & Webster, S. et al. (2020). Lockdown rollback checklist: Do countries meet WHO recommendations for rolling back lockdown? *Research Note,* Oxford Blavatnik School of Government, 1 May 2020, https://www.bsg.ox.ac.uk/sites/default/files/2020-05/2020-04-Lockdown-Rollback-Checklist-v2.pdf

Hamann, J. (2020). Germany: A balancing act between caution and exuberance amidst a crisis under control, in Robert Schuman Foundation (ed.), *Managing Covid-19, a journey through Europe,* 30 April 2020, pp. 22–4. https://www.robert-schuman.eu/en/doc/divers/FRS_seen_from_Germany.pdf

Hantrais, L. (2007). *Social policy in the European Union,* 3rd ed., London: Palgrave. https://www.macmillanihe.com/page/detail/Social-Policy-in-the-European-Union-Third-Edition/?K=9780230013094

Hantrais, L. (2009). *International comparative research: Theory, methods and practice,* London: Palgrave Macmillan. https://www.macmillanihe.com/page/detail/international-comparative-research-linda-hantrais/?k=9780230217683

Hantrais, L. (2019). *What Brexit means for EU and UK social policy,* Bristol: Policy Press. https://policy.bristoluniversitypress.co.uk/what-brexit-means-for-eu-and-uk-social-policy

Hantrais, L. (2020a). *Afterword: What Brexit and Covid-19 mean for EU and UK social policy,* Bristol: Policy Press. https://policy.bristoluniversitypress.co.uk/asset/8562/hantrais-online-afterword.pdf

Hantrais, L. (2020b). Comparing European reactions to Covid-19: Why policy decisions must be informed by reliable and contextualised evidence, *LSE EUROPP,* 19 May 2020. https://blogs.lse.ac.uk/europpblog/2020/05/19/comparing-european-reactions-to-covid-19-why-policy-decisions-must-be-informed-by-reliable-and-contextualised-evidence/

Henčeková, S. & Drugda, S. (2020). Change of government under COVID-19 emergency, *Verfassungsblog on matters constitutional,* 22 May 2020. https://verfassungsblog.de/slovakia-change-of-government-under-covid-19-emergency/

Henley, J. (2020). Coronavirus: EU states enact tough measures to stem spread, *The Guardian,* 10 March 2020. https://www.theguardian.com/world/2020/mar/10/coronavirus-several-eu-states-ban-mass-events-after-italian-lockdown

Hirsch, C. (2020). Europe's coronavirus lockdown measures compared, *Politico EU*, 15 April 2020. https://www.politico.eu/article/europes-coronavirus-lockdown-measures-compared/

House of Commons Library (2020). NHS staff from overseas: Statistics, *Research Briefing*, 4 June 2020. https://commonslibrary.parliament.uk/research-briefings/cbp-7783/

Institute for Government (2020). UK–EU future relationship: EU member state elections, *Explainers*, 30 April 2020. https://www.instituteforgovernment.org.uk/explainers/future-relationship-member-state-elections

Institut national d'études démographique (Ined) (2020). La démographie des décès par Covid-19. https://dc-covid.site.ined.fr/

Jaraczewski, J. (2020). An emergency by any other name? Measures against the COVID-19 pandemic in Poland, *Verfassungsblog on matters constitutional*, 24 April 2020. https://verfassungsblog.de/an-emergency-by-any-other-name-measures-against-the-covid-19-pandemic-in-poland/

Jürgensen, S. & Orlowski, F. (2020). Critique and crisis: The German struggle with pandemic control measures and the state of emergency, *Verfassungsblog on matters constitutional*, 19 April 2020. https://verfassungsblog.de/critique-and-crisis-the-german-struggle-with-pandemic-control-measures-and-the-state-of-emergency/

Karavokyris, G. (2020). The coronavirus crisis-law in Greece: A (constitutional) matter of life and death, *Verfassungsblog on matters constitutional*, 14 April 2020. https://verfassungsblog.de/the-coronavirus-crisis-law-in-greece-a-constitutional-matter-of-life-and-death/

Kovács, K. (2020). Hungary's Orbánistan: A complete arsenal of emergency powers, *Verfassungsblog on matters constitutional*, 6 April 2020. https://verfassungsblog.de/hungarys-orbanistan-a-complete-arsenal-of-emergency-powers/

Krelle, H., Barclay, C. & Tallack, C. (2020). Understanding excess mortality: What is the fairest way to compare COVID-19 deaths internationally? *The Health Foundation*. 6 May 2020. https://www.health.org.uk/news-and-comment/charts-and-infographics/understanding-excess-mortality-the-fairest-way-to-make-international-comparisons

Kupferschmidt, K. (2020). Why do some COVID-19 patients infect many others, whereas most don't spread the virus at all? *Science*, 19 May 2020. https://www.sciencemag.org/news/2020/05/why-do-some-covid-19-patients-infect-many-others-whereas-most-don-t-spread-virus-all

Laborderie, V. (2020). Belgium: Under the test of the coronavirus, in Robert Schuman Foundation (ed.), *Managing Covid-19, a journey through Europe*, 7 July 2020, pp. 7–11. https://www.robert-schuman.eu/en/doc/divers/Covid-19_Through_Europe.pdf

Lachmayer, K. (2020). Austria: Rule of law lacking in times of crisis, *Verfassungsblog on matters constitutional*, 28 Apr 2020. https://verfassungsblog.de/rule-of-law-lacking-in-times-of-crisis/

Laulhé Shaelou, S. & Manoli, A. (2020). A tale of two: The COVID-19 pandemic and the rule of law in Cyprus, *Verfassungsblog on matters constitutional*, 30 April 2020. https://verfassungsblog.de/a-tale-of-two-the-covid-19-pandemic-and-the-rule-of-law-in-cyprus/

Lebret, A. (2020). COVID-19 pandemic and derogation to human rights, *Journal of Law and the Biosciences*, 7(1), 1–15. https://doi.org/10.1093/jlb/lsaa015

Macek, L. (2020). *The East-West divide in the European Union in light of the COVID-19 crisis*, in Robert Schuman Foundation (ed.), *Managing Covid-19, a journey through Europe*, 7 July 2020, pp. 52–7. https://www.robert-schuman.eu/en/doc/divers/Covid-19_Through_Europe.pdf

Marmot, M., Allen, J., Boyce, T., Goldblatt, P. & Morrison, J. (2020). *Health equity in England: The Marmot review 10 years on*, London: Institute of Health Equity. https://www.health.org.uk/publications/reports/the-marmot-review-10-years-on

Maruste, R. (2020). State of emergency in Estonia, *Verfassungsblog on matters constitutional*, 17 May 2020. https://verfassungsblog.de/state-of-emergency-in-estonia/

Mathieson, K. (2020). Trust in scientists is eroding and we need to get it back. Transparency is more important than ever, *Telegraph*, 8 May 2020. https://www.telegraph.co.uk/global-health/science-and-disease/trust-scientists-eroding-need-get-back-transparency-important/

McGuirk, J. (2020). Pay up: Ireland will pay vastly more into new EU budget than it gets back, *GRIPT*, 21 July 2020. https://gript.ie/ireland-eu-budget-contribution-going-up/

Mock, J. (2020). Is herd immunity our best weapon again COVID-19? *Discover*, 4 May 2020. https://www.discovermagazine.com/health/is-herd-immunity-our-best-weapon-against-covid-19

Mutual Information System on Social Protection (MISSOC) (2020). MISSOC database. https://www.missoc.org/missoc-database/comparative-tables/

Neagu, B. (2020). Concerns raised over seasonal workers conditions in Germany, *Euractiv*, 22 April 2020. https://www.euractiv.com/section/agriculture-food/short_news/concerns-raised-over-seasonal-workers-conditions-in-germany/

OECD (2019a). *Health at a glance*, Paris: OECD Publishing. http://www.oecd.org/health/health-systems/health-at-a-glance-19991312.htm

OECD (2019b). *Recent trends in international migration of doctors, nurses and medical students*, Paris: OECD Publishing. DOI: 10.1787/5571ef48-en

OECD/European Union (2018). *Health at a glance: Europe 2018 state of health in the European cycle*, Paris: OECD Publishing. https://ec.europa.eu/health/state/glance_en

Oke, J. & Heneghan, C. (2020). Global COVID-19 case fatality rates, *Centre for Evidence-Based Medicine*, 17 March 2020. https://www.cebm.net/covid-19/global-covid-19-case-fatality-rates/

Our World in Data (n.d.). Research and data to make progress against the world's largest problems, *Coronavirus pandemic: Daily updated research and data*. https://ourworldindata.org/

Our World in Data (2020a). Case fatality rate vs total confirmed COVID-19 deaths, *Coronavirus pandemic: Daily updated research and data*. https://ourworldindata.org/grapher/deaths-covid-19-vs-case-fatality-rate?tab=table&time=2020-07-11

Our World in Data (2020b). Coronavirus (COVID-19) cases, *Statistics and research*. https://ourworldindata.org/covid-cases

Our World in Data (2020c). Coronavirus (COVID-19) deaths, *Statistics and research*. https://ourworldindata.org/covid-deaths

Oxford Blavatnik School of Government (n.d.a). *Oxford COVID-19 government response tracker*. https://covidtracker.bsg.ox.ac.uk/

Oxford Blavatnik School of Government (n.d.b). Relationship between number of Covid-19 cases and government response, *Oxford COVID-19 government response tracker*. https://covidtracker.bsg.ox.ac.uk/stringency-scatter

Papon, S. & Robert-Bobée, I. (2020). Une hausse des décès deux fois plus forte pour les personnes nées à l'étranger que pour celles nées en France en mars–avril 2020, *Insee Focus*, no. 198, 7 July 2020. https://www.insee.fr/fr/statistiques/4627049

Paun, C. (2020). Former French PM, health ministers to be investigated for pandemic response, *Politico EU*, 3 July 2020. https://www.politico.eu/article/former-french-pm-health-ministers-to-be-investigated-for-pandemic-response/

Petäistö, H. (2020). The corona virus will peak in Finland under the midnight sun, in Robert Schuman Foundation (ed.), *Managing Covid-19, a journey through Europe*, 16 April 2020, pp. 19–21. https://www.robert-schuman.eu/en/doc/divers/Covid-19_Through_Europe.pdf

Petersen, E., Koopmans, M., Go, U., Hamer, D.H., Petrosillo, N., Castelli, F. et al. (2020). Comparing SARS-CoV-2 with SARS-CoV and influenza pandemics, *Lancet, 20*(9), E238–E244. DOI: https://doi.org/10.1016/S1473-3099(20)30484-9

Petherick, A., Kira, B., Aymar, K., Hale, T., Phillips, T. & Webster, S. (2020). *Lockdown rollback checklist*, Oxford Blavatnik School of Government, 1 June 2020. https://www.bsg.ox.ac.uk/research/publications/lockdown-rollback-checklist

Platon, S. (2020). From one state of emergency to another – emergency powers in France, *Verfassungsblog on matters constitutional*, 9 April 2020. https://verfassungsblog.de/from-one-state-of-emergency-to-another-emergency-powers-in-france/

Platt, L. & Warwick, R. (2020). *Are some ethnic groups more vulnerable to COVID-19 than others?* Institute for Fiscal Studies, 1 May 2020. https://www.ifs.org.uk/inequality/chapter/are-some-ethnic-groups-more-vulnerable-to-covid-19-than-others/

Poenaru, F. & Rogozanu, C. (2020). Why social distancing 'doesn't apply' to Germany's migrant farmworkers, *Jacobin*, 23 May 2020. https://www.jacobinmag.com/2020/05/romanian-migrant-farmworkers-germany-european-union-corona virus

Politico EU (n.d.a). About us, *Politico EU*. https://www.politico.eu/about-us/

Politico EU (n.d.b). Coronavirus tracker, *Politico EU*. https://www.politico.eu/article/coronavirus-in-europe-by-the-numbers/

Politico EU (2020a). Europe's country-by-country travel restrictions explained, *Politico EU*, 31 July 2020. https://www.politico.eu/article/coronavirus-travel-europe-country-by-country-travel-restrictions-explained-summer-2020/

Politico EU (2020b). How Europe is responding to the coronavirus pandemic, *Politico EU*, 13 March 2020. https://www.politico.eu/article/how-europe-is-responding-to-the-coronavirus-pandemic/

Ritchie, H., Roser, M., Ortiz-Ospina, E. & Hasell, J. (2020). Excess mortality from the Coronavirus pandemic (COVID-19), *Coronavirus pandemic: Daily updated research and data*. https://ourworldindata.org/excess-mortality-covid

Republic of Poland (2020). Coronavirus: Information and recommendations, 16 April 2020. https://www.gov.pl/web/coronavirus/temporary-limitations

Robine, J-M. (2020). Coronavirus: Dans le champ de la mortalité, la sous-information est totale, pas seulement en France, *Le Monde*, 28 March 2020. https://www.lemonde.fr/planete/article/2020/03/28/coronavirus-dans-le-champ-de-la-mortalite-la-sous-information-est-totale-pas-seulement-en-france_6034773_3244.html

Sauer, B. (2020). Seen from Austria: As much freedom as possible, as many restrictions as necessary, in Robert Schuman Foundation (ed.), *Managing Covid-19, a journey through Europe*, 23 April 2020, pp. 3–6. https://www.robert-schuman.eu/en/doc/divers/Covid-19_Through_Europe.pdf

Scheinin, M. (2020). The COVID-19 emergency in Finland: Best practice and problems, *Verfassungsblog on matters constitutional*, 16 April 2020. https://verfassungs blog.de/the-covid-19-emergency-in-finland-best-practice-and-problems/

Selejan-Gutan, B. (2020). Romania in the Covid era: Between corona crisis and constitutional crisis, *Verfassungsblog on matters constitutional*, 21 May 2020. https://verfassungsblog.de/romania-in-the-covid-era-between-corona-crisis-and-constitutional-crisis/

Simmel, G. (1917). *Grundfragen der Soziologie (Individuum und Gesellschaft)*, 1st ed., Georg Simmel online, Berlin/Leipzig: G.J. Göschen. https://www.socio.ch/sim/grundfragen/grund_1.htm

Spiegelhalter, D. (2020). Coronavirus deaths: How does Britain compare with other countries? *The Guardian*, 30 April 2020. https://www.theguardian.com/comment isfree/2020/apr/30/coronavirus-deaths-how-does-britain-compare-with-other-countries?CMP=Share_iOSApp_Other

Statista (2020). Prevalence of diabetes in adult population in Europe 2019, by country, 24 June 2020. https://www.statista.com/statistics/1081006/prevalence-of-diabetes-in-europe/

Stoppioni, E. (2020). The protection of health must take precedence: Testing the constitutional state of crisis in Luxembourg, *Verfassungsblog on matters constitutional*, 29 April 2020. https://verfassungsblog.de/lithuanias-response-to-covid-19-quarantine-through-the-prism-of-human-rights-and-the-rule-of-law/

Tallack, C., Finch, D., Mihaylova, N., Barclay, C. & Watt, T. (2020). Understanding excess deaths: Variation in the impact of COVID-19 between countries, regions and localities, *The Health Foundation*, 4 June 2020. https://www.health.org.uk/news-and-comment/charts-and-infographics/understanding-excess-deaths-countries-regions-localities

Thijs, N., Hammerschmid, G. & Palaric, E. (2018). *A comparative overview of public administration characteristics and performance in EU28*, Luxembourg: Publications Office of the European Communities. https://ec.europa.eu/social/BlobServlet?docId=19208&langId=en

Triggle, N. (2020). Coronavirus: How to understand the death toll, *BBC News*, 16 April 2020. https://www.bbc.co.uk/news/health-51979654

UK Government Department for Education (2020). Guidance: Providing free school meals during the coronavirus (COVID-19) outbreak, 25 June 2020. https://www.gov.uk/government/publications/covid-19-free-school-meals-guidance/covid-19-free-school-meals-guidance-for-schools

UK Research and Innovation (UKRI) (2020). What is the purpose of testing for Covid-19? *Coronavirus: The science explained – UKRI*, 14 April 2020. https://corona virusexplained.ukri.org/en/article/vdt0006/

United Nations (2018). *World urbanization prospects: The 2018 revision*, Population Division, Department of Economic and Social Affairs, latest update 31 July 2020, New York: United Nations. https://population.un.org/wup/Download/Files/WUP 2018-F01-Total_Urban_Rural.xls

UN Global Health (2020). COVID-19: Emerging gender data and why it matters, *Women Count*, 26 June 2020. https://data.unwomen.org/resources/covid-19-emerging-gender-data-and-why-it-matters

Vassileva, R. (2020). Bulgaria: COVID-19 as an excuse to solidify autocracy? *Verfassungsblog on matters constitutional*, 10 April 2020. https://verfassungsblog.de/bulgaria-covid-19-as-an-excuse-to-solidify-autocracy/

Verbist, G., Diris, R. & Vandenbroucke (2020). Solidarity between generations in extended families: Old-age income as a way out of child poverty? *European Sociological Review, 36*(2), 317–32. DOI: https://doi.org/10.1093/esr/jcz052

Vikarská, Z. (2020). Czechs and balances – If the epidemiological situation allows..., *Verfassungsblog on matters constitutional*, 20 May 2020. https://verfassungsblog. de/right-restriction-or-restricting-rights-the-uk-acts-to-address-covid-19/

Violante, T. & Lanceiro, R.T. (2020). Coping with Covid-19 in Portugal: From constitutional normality to the state of emergency, *Verfassungsblog on matters constitutional*, 12 April 2020. https://verfassungsblog.de/coping-with-covid-19-in-portugal-from-constitutional-normality-to-the-state-of-emergency/

Vogel, G. (2020). How Sweden wasted a 'rare opportunity' to study coronavirus in schools, *Science*, 22 May 2020. https://www.sciencemag.org/news/2020/05/how-sweden-wasted-rare-opportunity-study-coronavirus-schools

Waterson, J. (2020). Public trust in UK government over coronavirus falls sharply, *The Guardian*, 1 June 2020. https://www.theguardian.com/world/2020/jun/01/public-trust-in-uk-government-over-coronavirus-falls-sharply

Wikipedia (n.d.a). List of European Union member states by political system. https://en.wikipedia.org/wiki/List_of_European_Union_member_states_by_political_system

Wikipedia (n.d.b). Pandemic by country and territory, *COVID-19 pandemic in Europe* https://en.wikipedia.org/wiki/COVID-19_pandemic_in_Europe#Statistics_by_country_and_territory

World Health Organisation (WHO) (n.d.a). Coronavirus disease (COVID-19) advice for the public. https://www.who.int/emergencies/diseases/novel-coronavirus-2019/advice-for-public

World Health Organisation (WHO) (n.d.b). Definitions: mortality rate, *Humanitarian Health Action*. https://www.who.int/hac/about/definitions/en/

World Health Organisation (WHO) (2009). *WHO guidelines on hand hygiene in health care*, Geneva: WHO. https://apps.who.int/iris/bitstream/handle/10665/44102/9789241597906_eng.pdf;jsessionid=E5B2B39987CF96C726EC64D59A2C8CEC?sequence=1

World Health Organisation (WHO) (2020a). Recommendations to member states to improve hand hygiene practices to help prevent the transmission of the COVID-19 virus: Interim guidance, 1 April 2020. https://apps.who.int/iris/rest/bitstreams/1273865/retrieve

World Health Organisation (WHO) (2020b). Q&A: Masks and COVID-19, 7 June 2020. https://www.who.int/emergencies/diseases/novel-coronavirus-2019/question-and-answers-hub/q-a-detail/q-a-on-covid-19-and-masks

World Health Organisation (WHO) (2020c). WHO campaigns: Year of the Nurse and the Midwife, March 2020. https://www.who.int/campaigns/year-of-the-nurse-and-the-midwife-2020

World Health Organisation (WHO) (2020d). WHO Director-General's opening remarks at the media briefing on COVID-19, 13 March 2020. https://www.who.int/dg/speeches/detail/who-director-general-s-opening-remarks-at-the-mission-briefing-on-covid-19---13-march-2020

World Obesity (2020). Coronavirus (COVID-19) & obesity. https://www.worldobesity.org/news/statement-coronavirus-covid-19-obesity

Worldometer (n.d.a). About Worldometer. https://www.worldometers.info/coronavirus/about/#about

Worldometer (n.d.b). COVID-19 reported cases and deaths by country, territory, or conveyance. https://www.worldometers.info/coronavirus/?referer=app

Worldometer (n.d.c). Definitions. https://www.worldometers.info/coronavirus/about/#definitions

World Population Review (2020). Obesity rates by country. https://worldpopulation review.com/country-rankings/obesity-rates-by-country

Zagorc, S. & Bardutzky, S. (2020). Business as usual, but to the unusual extremes: Slovenia and Covid-19, *Verfassungsblog on matters constitutional*, 26 April 2020, https://verfassungsblog.de/business-as-usual-but-to-the-unusual-extremes-slovenia-and-covid-19/

Index